EMPOWER LIGHT

*Sustainable Weight Loss &
Health for Women*

MUJAHID BAKHT

1

EBook ISBN: 979-8-89302-062-5

Paperback ISBN: 979-8-89302-060-1

Hardcover ISBN: 979-8-89302-061-8

Published By:

ATLAS AMAZON, LLC.

244 Fifth Avenue, D210, New York, N.Y.

United States of America

SECOND EDITION

TABLE OF CONTENTS

ABOUT THE AUTHOR

LIFE HISTORY: Mr. Bakhtis a mature, experienced, excessively enthusiastic, energetic administrator with thirty-eight years of proven experience as a businessman in international marketing and public relations. Mr. Bakht is an International Real Estate Specialist and Professional Business and Projects Consultant and Advisor. He was born in Pakistan and educated in Pakistan and the USA. Presently, American Citizen belongs to a business-oriented family. Thirty-eight years Resident of New York, USA.

BUSINESS HISTORY: Mr. Bakht is a Founder and President of Atlas Amazon, LLC., Mr. Bakht is a business developer and multilingual business specialist in the Caribbean, South East Asia, and the Middle East emerging markets Mr. Bakht has served, met, and hosted many heads of the States. Also, maintain a close relationship with investors of high net worth in the USA.

CAREER: Mr. Bakht has been engaged with many multinational companies in the fields of international real estate investment, communication, technology, diamond, gold, mining, Pre-Feb housing, wind and solar energy, outsourcing management, and project consulting, along with business partners and associates worldwide. Mr. Bakht has participated in major national and international conferences, including participated in United Nations (U.N.O.) conferences.

TRAVEL: Mr. Bakht is well-traveled and has visited many countries around the world.

MANAGEMENT EXPERIENCE: Thirty-eight years of diversified experience in project consulting, marketing, and business management. As a Director of Marketing, Director of Public Relations, Director of International Affairs, Executive Vice President, President, CEO, and Chairman of many national and multinational companies. Mr. Bakht hired and trained many professionals as business consultants in international marketing and supervised them.

CERTIFICATE OF ACHIEVEMENT: The Achievement Award was presented to Mr. Bakht by Stephen Fossler for five years of continued growth and customer satisfaction from 1996 to 2001.

HONORS MEMBER:Madison Who's Who of Professionals, having demonstrated exemplary achievement and distinguished contributions to the business community, registered at the Library of Congress in Washington D.C. USA. (2007 and 2008)

HONORS MEMBER: Premiere Who's Who International, professional business executive having demonstrated exemplary achievement and distinguished contributions to the International business community, 2008 and 2009.

CERTIFICATES: Certificate of Authenticity from Bill Rodham Clinton, President of the United States, and Hillary Rodham Clinton First Lady, USA. (July 20, 2000);

CERTIFICATE OF AUTHENTICITY: from Terence R. McAuliffe, Chairman of Democratic National Committee,

Tom Dachle, Senate Democratic Leader, Dick Gephardt, House Democratic Leader, USA. (June 16, 2001);

CERTIFICATE OF AUTHENTICITY: from Terence R. McAuliffe, Chairman of Democratic National Committee, USA. (April 16, 2002).

CHAPTER 1

The Realities of Weight Loss Today

———— ✕ ————

Conflicting advice, big promises, and endless trends often surround the topic of weight loss. For many women, it can feel like every new diet or fitness fad guarantees fast results, only to leave them feeling disappointed or overwhelmed. The truth is, successful weight loss is not about chasing shortcuts or following the latest craze. Instead, it requires a realistic understanding of what actually works for women in the real world.

In this chapter, we examine why many diets fail, why quick fixes rarely last, and how misleading ideas can complicate the process more than necessary. We'll explore what sets real, lasting change apart from temporary results and set the stage for a healthier approach, one based on facts, patience, and confidence in your ability to succeed.

Why most diets fail women

Many women start new diets with hope and determination, only to find themselves back at square one a few weeks or months later. This cycle is frustrating, and it's more common than most people realize. One primary reason is that most diets are designed as one-size-fits-all solutions. They fail to account for women's unique hormonal changes, body types, and the realities of everyday life. Strict calorie limits and food restrictions may yield results initially, but they often leave women feeling deprived, tired, and stressed.

Another reason diets fail is that they rarely address the emotional and social sides of eating. Life is full of celebrations, stress, and busy days, and a rigid meal plan can be hard to follow when things get hectic. When willpower wanes or something unexpected occurs, old habits tend to resurface.

Quick-fix diets can slow down metabolism and lead to muscle loss, making it even more challenging to maintain weight loss in the long run. True success comes from building habits you can stick with and learning how to adapt to real-life challenges, not from chasing short-term results.

Unpacking the culture of quick fixes

Today's weight loss industry thrives on promises of fast results and dramatic transformations. Social media, advertisements, and celebrity endorsements often showcase stories of overnight success, with claims that you can drop several dress sizes in just a few weeks. These messages are everywhere, and they can make slow, steady progress feel dull or even like failure. The truth is, this culture of quick fixes often does more harm than good.

Many women are drawn to programs that promise rapid weight loss because they tap into our desire for immediate change. It's natural to want results as soon as possible, especially if you've been struggling for a long time.

Unfortunately, these promises rarely match reality. Most rapid weight loss plans involve extreme calorie restriction, cutting out entire food groups, or relying on expensive supplements. While they may show quick changes on the scale, these results are usually short-lived.

The primary issue with quick fixes is that they overlook how the body truly functions. Rapid weight loss can lead to muscle loss, lower metabolism, and even nutritional deficiencies. Your body is designed to protect you from starvation, so extreme diets can trigger a survival response, making it harder to lose weight the next time you try. Even worse, many people regain all the weight they lost and sometimes even more once they return to their regular eating habits.

There's also an emotional cost to this cycle. Constantly starting and stopping diets can damage your confidence and make you feel like you've failed, when in fact, the problem was with the diet itself, not with you. This mindset can lead to guilt, shame, and a negative relationship with food, turning weight loss into a stressful experience instead of a positive journey.

Quick fixes might look appealing on the surface, but they don't teach you the skills needed for long-term success. Real progress comes from building better habits, understanding your body, and learning how to make healthy choices in everyday life. When you step away from the culture of instant results and give yourself time to change, you set yourself up for something much more valuable: a healthier, happier life that lasts.

How to spot weight loss myths

The world of weight loss is filled with advice, much of which is misleading or simply untrue. Spotting the myths early can save you time, money, and frustration. One of the first signs of a weight loss myth is a promise that sounds too good to be true. Claims of losing significant amounts of weight in just days or without any effort should raise a red flag. Genuine, healthy weight loss always takes time and consistency.

Another common sign is advice that encourages extreme restrictions. Diets that require you to eliminate entire food groups, restrict you to eating only one type of food, or prohibit meals altogether are rarely safe or effective. Your body needs a variety of nutrients to function optimally, and overly strict rules can make eating a stressful and unsustainable experience.

Be cautious of products or plans that rely on "miracle" ingredients or supplements. No pill, powder, or tea can replace a balanced diet and healthy habits. These products often come with big promises but little real evidence to support them.

Be cautious of advice that overlooks your unique needs. Any plan that treats everyone the same, regardless of age, health, or lifestyle, fails to recognize how different bodies work. True, lasting change comes from solutions that fit your circumstances.

Look for information that lacks credible sources. Reliable advice is backed by science, not just testimonials or flashy before-and-after photos. Always verify the source of the information and don't hesitate to ask questions or consult a qualified professional.

By learning to spot these myths, you protect yourself from disappointment and stay focused on what really works. Remember, there are no shortcuts, but with the proper knowledge, you can make choices that truly support your health and well-being.

Rewriting your personal story

Everyone has a history with weight loss, full of past attempts, ups and downs, and maybe even moments of frustration or self-doubt. But your past does not define your future. Rewriting your personal story means letting go of old labels, judgments, and the idea that you are somehow destined to struggle forever.

It starts with seeing yourself in a new light. Instead of focusing on what went wrong before, shift your attention to what you've learned along the way. Every setback is a chance to grow wiser and stronger. Maybe you discovered what doesn't work for your body, or you realised how stress and emotions play a bigger role than you thought. These lessons are valuable building blocks, not failures.

Changing your story also means treating yourself with more kindness and respect. It's easy to fall into negative self-talk, especially if you feel stuck or discouraged. But positive change comes when you believe you are capable of something better. Remind yourself of your strengths and the progress you've made, no matter how small it seems.

Most importantly, rewriting your story is about taking control, one step at a time. You get to decide what health means for you, not anyone else. As you move forward, focus on choices and habits that match your real life and goals. Over time, these new chapters will add up to a story you can truly be proud of — one built on growth, resilience, and genuine success.

What sustainable success really means

Sustainable success in weight loss isn't about a number on the scale or how quickly you reach your goal. It's about building habits that fit your real life and last for years, not just weeks. When you focus on sustainability, you're choosing a path that supports your health, your energy, and your happiness day after day.

This success means making changes you can actually stick with, like finding ways to enjoy healthy meals, moving your body in ways that feel good, and allowing yourself some flexibility along the way. It's not about perfection or following strict rules, but about progress and patience.

Sustainable success also means looking beyond short-term results. Instead of celebrating quick fixes, you start to value how much stronger, more confident, and more capable you feel as your habits improve. You learn how to handle setbacks without giving up and how to keep moving forward, even on the most challenging days.

21

True, lasting change happens when healthy choices become a natural part of your routine. It's about feeling better in your body, having more energy for the things you love, and knowing that you're caring for yourself in a way that works long term. That's the real meaning of success, and it's something worth aiming for.

The first step: mindset

Before making changes to your diet or starting a new exercise plan, the most crucial place to begin is with your mindset. How you think about weight loss can shape your entire experience. If you approach your journey with harsh self-criticism or focus only on what you want to "fix," progress often feels more challenging and less rewarding.

A healthy mindset is rooted in patience, self-respect, and the belief that positive change is possible, regardless of your starting point. Instead of seeing healthy habits as a punishment or restriction, try to view them as acts of self-care. Celebrate your efforts and any minor improvements, rather than waiting until you hit a specific target to feel proud.

It's also helpful to expect ups and downs along the way. Setbacks are normal, but they don't mean you've failed. With the right mindset, challenges become opportunities to learn and adjust. Each day is a fresh start, and your thoughts can be one of your most excellent tools for long-term success.

When your mindset is focused on growth, self-compassion, and steady progress, every step forward feels more achievable, and a healthier life becomes something you genuinely believe you can reach.

CHAPTER 2

Understanding Your Unique Physiology

No two women are exactly alike, and that includes how each body responds to food, exercise, and stress. Many weight loss plans ignore these differences and offer generic advice, but your journey should reflect your own unique needs. Understanding how your body works, its strengths, rhythms, and challenges, gives you a real advantage.

In this chapter, we'll examine the key factors that shape your metabolism, the role hormones play, and why both genetics and lifestyle matter. You'll learn how to listen to your body's signals and make decisions that are truly right for you. When you know what makes you unique, it's easier to set realistic goals and find strategies that actually work in your everyday life.

What makes your body unique?

Every woman's body has its own story, shaped by genetics, lifestyle, and personal history. These differences influence how you gain or lose weight, how your energy levels fluctuate, and even how you respond to certain foods or types of exercise. For example, some women notice that their bodies hold onto weight in certain areas, while others may see changes more quickly.

Your metabolism, the rate at which your body uses energy, can also vary based on factors such as age, muscle mass, hormones, and even your daily routine. Medical history, sleep patterns, and stress also play a role. What works for one person may not be the best approach for someone else.

Understanding and accepting these differences is the first step in making lasting changes. Rather than comparing yourself to others or following a plan that doesn't fit your lifestyle, take time to notice what makes your body feel its best. When you recognize your strengths and needs, you can set more realistic goals and build a healthy routine that truly fits you.

Female metabolism basics

Metabolism is the process your body uses to turn food into energy. For women, metabolism is influenced by several unique factors, including hormones, age, and body composition. Generally, women tend to have a slightly slower metabolism compared to men, primarily due to differences in muscle mass and natural hormonal fluctuations.

Muscle burns more calories than fat, even at rest, so women with more lean muscle may notice their bodies use energy more efficiently. However, natural changes such as puberty, pregnancy, or menopause can all impact how your metabolism functions over time.

Eating too little or skipping meals can actually slow your metabolism, making it harder to lose weight and increasing your likelihood of feeling tired. Instead, balanced meals with sufficient protein, healthy fats, and complex carbohydrates help maintain a steady metabolism and boost energy levels.

Physical activity also plays an important role. Regular movement, especially strength training, supports a healthier metabolism by helping you build or maintain muscle. Listening to your body and nourishing it well is the best way to support your metabolism, no extreme diets or shortcuts needed.

Hormones and weight management

Hormones are chemical messengers in your body that control many processes, including how you gain, lose, or store weight. For women, hormonal balance is crucial because even slight changes can have a noticeable impact on appetite, cravings, and energy levels.

Estrogen, progesterone, insulin, and cortical are just a few hormones that play a part in weight management. For example, estrogen levels fluctuate during the menstrual cycle, pregnancy, or menopause, which can alter how your body stores fat or affect your appetite. High levels of the stress hormone cortical, often triggered by lack of sleep or chronic worry, can make it easier to hold onto weight, especially around the middle.

Insulin, which helps regulate blood sugar levels, can also influence how your body utilizes or stores energy. When insulin levels are out of balance, it becomes more challenging to lose weight or resist cravings for sugary foods.

Understanding the role hormones play means paying attention to patterns in your body. If you notice regular changes in your appetite, mood, or weight, it may be connected to your hormones. Healthy habits, such as balanced meals, regular physical activity, and adequate sleep, can help stabilize your hormones, making weight management less of a struggle. If things feel out of balance for a long time, talking with your doctor can also be helpful.

Genetics vs. habits

When it comes to weight management, both genetics and daily habits play essential roles. Genetics can influence factors such as body shape, weight gain and loss, and the location of fat storage. These inherited traits are passed down from your family and set a starting point for your health journey.

However, your habits, including what you eat, how active you are, how you manage stress, and how much you sleep, also have a powerful impact. While you can't change your genes, you do have control over the choices you make every day. Even small changes in habits can lead to noticeable improvements over time, regardless of your starting point.

Some people may feel discouraged if they have a family history of weight struggles, but your genes do not decide your future alone. Healthy habits can help you optimize your unique body and make it easier to manage your weight in a way that suits you. Focusing on what you can change, rather than what you can't, puts you in charge of your progress.

Tracking progress safely

Keeping track of your progress can help you stay motivated and see the results of your efforts. However, it's important to use healthy and realistic methods that support your overall well-being. While many people focus only on the number on the scale, actual progress can be measured in many ways.

Consider tracking how your clothes fit, your energy levels, or improvements in your strength and stamina. Taking occasional body measurements, noting changes in sleep quality, or keeping a simple journal about your mood and confidence can all provide valuable feedback.

Weighing yourself too often or becoming overly focused on small changes can lead to frustration. Try to check in with yourself once a week, or even less frequently, and remember that daily fluctuations in weight are normal. Use progress photos or written notes to look back and see your long-term journey, rather than just focusing on day-to-day shifts.

Most importantly, tracking should feel encouraging, not stressful. Celebrate small wins, like making healthier choices or sticking to a new routine. By using safe and positive ways to monitor your progress, you keep your focus on building habits that last, rather than chasing quick results.

Adapting to life stages

Your body's needs and abilities can change over time, especially as you move through different life stages. Hormonal shifts, aging, pregnancy, menopause, or changes in your daily routine can all impact how you gain or lose weight and how your body feels on a day-to-day basis.

It's essential to recognize that what worked for you in your twenties may not be the best approach in your forties or fifties. For example, building or maintaining muscle becomes more critical as you age, while metabolism may slow down due to age or hormonal changes. Times of high stress, major life events, or family responsibilities may also require you to adjust your approach to meals, movement, or self-care.

The key is to stay flexible and open to making changes as needed. Listen to your body and adjust your habits to match your current needs, rather than relying on past routines. Seek advice from health professionals when you face new challenges or notice significant shifts. By being patient with yourself and willing to adapt, you make it easier to stay healthy and feel good through every stage of life.

CHAPTER 3

Emotional Health & Sustainable Change

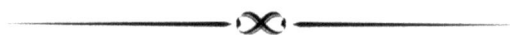

--- ∞ ---

Lasting weight loss is about more than food choices or workout routines; it's also deeply connected to your emotional health. How you handle stress, manage emotions, and respond to life's challenges can shape your relationship with eating, movement, and self-care. Many women find that moments of frustration, sadness, or anxiety lead to habits that get in the way of their goals.

This chapter explores the profound connection between your emotions and your ability to bring about significant, lasting changes. You'll learn how to recognize triggers, develop healthy ways to cope, and build a stronger sense of self-worth. By caring for your emotional well-being, you establish a strong foundation for lasting changes that not only benefit you but also improve your overall well-being in every aspect of your life.

Emotional triggers for overeating

For many women, eating is about more than just satisfying hunger. Emotions like stress, boredom, loneliness, or even happiness can lead to reaching for food as a source of comfort or distraction. These emotional triggers are a regular part of life, but if they happen often, they can make weight loss feel much harder.

It's common to use food as a way to cope with complex emotions or to reward yourself after a challenging day. Certain situations, such as arguments, work pressure, or feeling left out, might set off cravings for snacks or sweets, even if you're not physically hungry. Sometimes, just the habit of eating while watching TV or scrolling through your phone can become a way to soothe emotions without realizing it.

The first step in overcoming emotional overeating is learning to recognize your triggers. Start paying attention to when and why you feel the urge to eat outside of regular meals. Are there specific times of day, people, or situations that trigger it? Once you understand what triggers these habits, you can start developing healthier responses, such as taking a walk, journaling, or simply pausing to check in with yourself. Understanding your emotional triggers is an essential part of building a more balanced and mindful relationship with food.

Stress, sleep, and weight

The way you handle stress and the quality of your sleep can have a significant impact on your weight. When stress builds up, your body produces more of the hormone cortical, which can increase cravings for comfort foods and make it easier to store fat, especially around your waist. High stress levels can also make it harder to find the motivation to exercise or prepare healthy meals.

Sleep also plays a key role. Not getting enough rest can disrupt the hormones that control hunger and fullness, often leading to overeating or late-night snacking. Lack of sleep can also drain your energy, making you more likely to skip workouts or reach for quick, unhealthy options when you're tired.

Managing stress with healthy habits, such as gentle movement, talking with friends, or spending time in nature, can help keep your body's responses in balance. Prioritizing good sleep by maintaining a regular schedule and creating a calm bedtime routine also supports your weight loss efforts. When you take care of your stress and sleep, it becomes much easier to stick with your healthy choices and feel better each day.

Building resilience against emotional eating

Emotional eating is a typical response to life's challenges, but it doesn't have to control your journey. Building resilience means developing the inner strength to handle stress, sadness, or frustration without automatically turning to food for comfort. This is not about having perfect willpower; instead, it's about learning new ways to support yourself when emotions run high.

Start by paying attention to your emotional patterns. Notice when you tend to crave certain foods and what might be happening in your life at those times. Sometimes, simply pausing to ask yourself if you're truly hungry or if you're feeling bored, anxious, or upset can break the automatic cycle. Keeping a small journal or jotting notes in your phone about your feelings before eating can help you spot trends and triggers.

Once you become more aware of your patterns, you can experiment with healthier coping strategies. If you find yourself reaching for snacks during stressful moments, try stepping outside for some fresh air, calling a friend, or practicing a few deep breaths. Even short walks or gentle stretching can shift your mood and give your mind a chance to reset. The key is to find what works for you, activities that bring real relief and comfort, rather than just a temporary distraction.

Another essential part of resilience is self-compassion. It's normal to slip up sometimes, especially when life feels overwhelming. Instead of blaming yourself or giving up, remind yourself that change takes time and persistence. Speak to yourself the way you would comfort a close friend: with understanding, encouragement, and patience.

Setting small, realistic goals can also help you build confidence. Celebrate progress, whether it's choosing a healthy snack over sweets or acknowledging your feelings before eating. Over time, these small victories add up and make it easier to stay on track, even during stressful periods.

Remember that you don't have to do it all alone. Reaching out for support from friends, family, or a professional can make a big difference. By developing healthy ways to manage your emotions and being gentle with yourself when you struggle, you create a solid foundation for lasting, positive change. Resilience is not about never having tough days; it's about finding the strength to keep moving forward, no matter what comes your way.

Sleep hygiene for weight loss

Getting enough restful sleep is often overlooked when it comes to weight loss, but it plays a significant role in your success. A good night's sleep helps balance the hormones that regulate hunger and fullness, making it easier to avoid overeating and manage cravings. When you're well-rested, you're more likely to have steady energy, a better mood, and the motivation to stick with healthy habits.

Sleep hygiene refers to establishing routines and an environment that promotes high-quality rest. Try to keep a regular sleep schedule by going to bed and waking up at the same time each day, even on weekends. Limit caffeine and heavy meals close to bedtime, as they can make it harder to fall asleep. Creating a relaxing nighttime routine, such as reading, gentle stretching, or listening to calming music, can help signal to your body that it's time to wind down.

Keep your bedroom dark, quiet, and calm, and put away screens at least thirty minutes before bed. The blue light from phones and TVs can disrupt your body's natural sleep cycle. If you wake up during the night, try to stay calm and focus on slow, deep breathing until you drift back to sleep.

Making sleep a priority is just as important as nutrition and exercise. When your body gets the rest it needs, you're better prepared to make healthy choices, handle stress, and see steady progress on your weight loss journey.

The power of self-image

How you see yourself can shape your progress far more than you might realize. Self-image is the collection of thoughts and beliefs you hold about your own body, abilities, and worth. When your self-image is positive, you're more likely to treat yourself with care, set realistic goals, and bounce back from setbacks.

A negative self-image, on the other hand, can make healthy changes feel like punishment or seem unattainable. You may find yourself focusing only on flaws or comparing your journey to others, which can undermine your confidence and motivation. Over time, these patterns can hinder progress and make it more challenging to maintain new habits.

Building a better self-image starts with shifting your focus from criticism to appreciation. Notice your strengths and celebrate small victories, whether it's making a healthier meal choice or taking a short walk. Speak to yourself with the same respect and kindness you would offer a close friend. Remember, your worth isn't defined by a number on the scale or anyone else's opinion.

As you work toward your goals, a positive self-image becomes a powerful ally. It helps you approach challenges with resilience and opens the door to lasting, meaningful change because you believe you're truly worth the effort.

Tools to break old patterns

Breaking old habits isn't easy, but the right tools can make the process smoother and more successful. The first step is awareness; notice when and why certain habits appear. Keeping a simple journal or using a habit-tracking app can help you spot patterns in your eating, exercise, or self-care routines.

Planning is another powerful tool. Prepare healthy snacks in advance, schedule regular activity into your day, or set gentle reminders for mindful moments. These small actions can help you make better choices, even on busy or stressful days.

Replacing old habits with new, positive ones is key. If you tend to snack when you're bored, try taking a quick walk or calling a friend instead. If stress makes you reach for sweets, experiment with deep breathing, stretching, or a relaxing activity you enjoy. Over time, these new responses can become your go-to habits.

Support also matters. Share your goals with a trusted friend or family member, or join a supportive community online or in person. Accountability can help you stay motivated and remind you that you're not alone in making changes.

Be patient with yourself. Breaking old patterns takes time and practice. Celebrate progress, forgive slip-ups, and continue to look for small steps forward. Each healthy choice builds your confidence and moves you closer to lasting change.

Seeking support when needed

Lasting change is rarely a solo journey. Even the most determined people can face challenges, setbacks, or moments of doubt along the way. Seeking support is not a sign of weakness; it's a practical step that increases the likelihood of success and makes the process less stressful.

Support can come in many forms. It might be a friend who listens without judgment, a family member who accompanies you on a walk, or a group of people with similar goals who share ideas and offer encouragement. Professional guidance from a dietitian, fitness coach, or counselor can offer clarity and motivation when you feel stuck.

Reaching out for support gives you the chance to learn from others and feel less alone on your journey. It can provide new ideas, help you see problems from a fresh perspective, or offer a reminder that setbacks are a common occurrence. If you find yourself struggling, don't hesitate to ask for help, whether that means joining a class, finding an online community, or just having an honest conversation with someone you trust.

Real strength lies in knowing when to lean on others. Accepting support, sharing your experiences, and giving encouragement in return can make your path to better health smoother and more rewarding.

CHAPTER 4

Laying the Foundation for Success

———— ⋊⋉ ————

Real, lasting change begins with a strong foundation. Before jumping into strict diets or intense workout plans, it's essential to set yourself up for success with clear goals, a supportive environment, and practical strategies that work for your life. The habits and routines you build now will carry you through challenges and help you stay on track, even when motivation dips.

In this chapter, you'll discover how to set meaningful goals, identify obstacles before they arise, and create an environment that supports your journey. By taking the time to lay this groundwork, you give yourself the best chance for steady progress and long-term results, turning healthy choices into a natural part of your everyday life.

Setting realistic, inspiring goals

Setting goals is one of the most important steps you can take on your weight loss journey, but not all goals are created equal. Many people begin with broad, vague intentions, such as "lose weight" or "get fit," but these goals can quickly feel overwhelming or unclear. Real progress comes from setting goals that are both realistic and inspiring, goals that encourage you to move forward while also respecting where you are right now.

A realistic goal is specific and achievable. Instead of aiming to "lose a lot of weight fast," focus on what you can do in a healthy, steady way, like aiming to lose one or two pounds a week. Break bigger goals into smaller steps, such as walking for twenty minutes each day or adding an extra serving of vegetables to your meals. These smaller milestones are easier to achieve and provide you with regular moments of success to celebrate.

Goals are most potent when they are meaningful to you. Think about why you want to make changes, not just for a number on the scale, but for deeper reasons like having more energy to play with your children, feeling stronger at work, or being able to travel comfortably. Connecting your goals to your values keeps you motivated, especially on days when progress feels slow.

Write down your goals and review them regularly. Seeing your intentions in writing gives them weight and reminds you of your commitment. Some people find it helpful to post their goals in a visible location, such as on the fridge or a bathroom mirror. You may also want to share your goals with a trusted friend or family member for added accountability and encouragement.

That flexibility is part of success. Life is unpredictable, and sometimes you'll need to adjust your goals to fit new circumstances. If a goal starts to feel out of reach, it's okay to make changes. What matters most is that you keep moving forward in a way that feels manageable and positive.

Celebrate every step, no matter how small. Each healthy choice, each day you stick to your plan, is a sign of progress. When you set realistic, inspiring goals, you build a path that is steady, rewarding, and truly your own. This is how real change begins and how it lasts.

Building your weight loss roadmap

A successful journey needs more than just good intentions; it requires a plan. Building your weight loss roadmap means outlining the steps you'll take, identifying your resources, and deciding how you'll handle challenges along the way. This plan doesn't have to be complicated. In fact, the best roadmaps are straightforward, flexible, and focused on your real life.

Start by defining your primary goal and the timeframe you're aiming for. Next, break your big goal into smaller, manageable steps. These steps might include improving your breakfast, adding a few walks each week, or getting to bed on time. Each step brings you closer to your goal and provides you with a specific area to focus on.

A good roadmap also considers your schedule, preferences, and possible obstacles. Think about busy days, social events, or times you usually struggle, and decide ahead of time how you'll respond. Planning for these situations keeps you prepared and reduces the chance of getting off track.

Here's an example of how you might organize your plan:

Goal	Action Step	Timeline	How I'll Track Progress
Lose 8 pounds in 2 months	Walk 20 minutes after dinner, 5 days a week	Start this week	Mark on calendar
Eat more vegetables	Add a serving to lunch and dinner	Ongoing	Daily food log
Reduce sugary drinks	Replace with water or herbal tea	Start today	Count servings each day
Improve sleep routine	Go to bed by 10:30 p.m. nightly	This month	Bedtime journal

Review your roadmap often. Adjust your steps if something isn't working or if you reach a new milestone. This process is about steady progress, not perfection.

Remember to include rewards and celebrations in your plan. Recognize your achievements, whether it's sticking to your walking routine for a week or choosing a healthy snack during a busy day. By building a roadmap that fits your life, you provide yourself with a clear and encouraging guide to follow, making it much easier to reach your goals.

Creating a positive environment

Your surroundings play a decisive role in shaping your habits and supporting your goals. Creating a positive environment means making small changes at home, at work, and even in your social circles that help you stay on track with your weight loss journey.

Start with your kitchen. Keep healthy foods visible and easily accessible. Wash and cut vegetables ahead of time, place fruit on the counter, and store snacks, such as nuts or yogurt, where you'll see them first. At the same time, limit the presence of tempting, less nutritious options by placing them out of sight or reducing their frequency of purchase.

Consider your daily routines as well. Set reminders to drink water, leave your walking shoes by the door, or schedule exercise time on your calendar. The easier you make healthy choices, the more likely you are to stick with them.

The people around you matter as well. Let friends and family know about your goals so they can offer encouragement and even join in. Spend more time with those who support your efforts and less time in situations where you feel pressured to break your routine.

A positive environment is also about your mindset. Fill your space with uplifting reminders such as motivational quotes, progress photos, or a journal where you note your successes. Celebrate your achievements, no matter how small, and be gentle with yourself if you have a tough day.

Shaping your environment to make healthy habits easier sets you up for greater success and makes your journey more enjoyable and sustainable.

Identifying obstacles before they happen

Every weight loss journey comes with its share of challenges, but being prepared can make a big difference. Identifying obstacles before they happen helps you respond with confidence, rather than feeling caught off guard. This proactive approach enables you to create a plan for moments when your routine is challenged.

Start by thinking about past experiences. Were there specific times when you found it hard to stick with healthy habits, like during holidays, late-night cravings, or after a stressful day at work? Write down these situations and consider what typically gets in the way, whether it's a busy schedule, social pressure, or simply feeling tired.

Once you've listed your common obstacles, brainstorm solutions in advance. If you know evenings are tough, prepare healthy snacks or meals ahead of time to make them easier. If social events tempt you to overeat, decide what you'll enjoy in moderation and have a strategy for saying no to extras. For days when motivation is low, keep a short workout video or walk planned as a backup.

It also helps to communicate your goals to those around you, so they understand your choices and can offer support rather than extra temptation. Maintaining a positive environment and setting reminders can help you avoid common pitfalls.

Obstacles are a regular part of any change. By planning for them before they happen, you turn challenges into opportunities to practice new skills and build resilience. This mindset keeps you moving forward, even when the journey doesn't go exactly as planned.

Finding accountability that works for you

Accountability can make a big difference when you're trying to reach your weight loss goals. Knowing that someone or something is tracking your progress helps you stay focused, motivated, and more likely to follow through, especially on days when your willpower feels low.

Accountability comes in many forms, so it's essential to find what fits your personality and lifestyle. For some people, sharing their goals with a trusted friend or family member provides encouragement and honest feedback. Others benefit from joining a group or online community where members support one another and celebrate successes together.

Journaling or using a tracking app can also be a powerful tool. Writing down your meals, workouts, or moods creates a sense of responsibility towards yourself and allows you to see patterns or progress over time. Some people set up regular check-ins with a coach or mentor, while others use reminders or rewards as a form of motivation.

Choose the method that feels natural and comfortable for you. If one approach doesn't work, don't hesitate to try another. The key is to have a system that helps you reflect on your choices, celebrate successes, and learn from any setbacks.

No matter how you do it, accountability keeps you honest with yourself and helps you stay connected to your goals. With the proper support in place, you're much more likely to keep moving forward and make lasting, positive changes.

Staying motivated beyond week 1

The excitement of starting something new can carry you through the first few days, but maintaining motivation after the initial rush fades is often a challenge. To keep moving forward, it's essential to find ways to stay inspired and committed, even when the journey feels less exciting or progress slows down.

Start by reminding yourself why you began. Keeping your main reasons and goals visible, whether on a sticky note, in your phone, or in a journal, can help you stay connected to your purpose. Reflect on the benefits you're already noticing, like better sleep, more energy, or feeling proud of your efforts.

Break your big goals into smaller milestones and celebrate each one as you achieve them. Completing a week of regular walks, cooking a new healthy meal, or saying no to extra sweets at an event are all victories worth acknowledging. These small successes build confidence and create a positive feedback loop that keeps you motivated.

Stay flexible and patient with yourself. Progress is rarely a straight line, and it's normal to have good and bad days. Instead of focusing only on the result, pay attention to the habits you're building and the effort you're putting in.

Connect with supportive people who understand your journey. Share your challenges and achievements, and let their encouragement help you keep going. Motivation will ebb and flow, but with the right mindset and support, you'll find it much easier to stick with your healthy changes over time.

Small wins and lasting confidence

Significant milestones don't just measure success in weight loss; they're built on small wins achieved day after day. These small victories might seem minor at first, but they add up and help you create new habits that last. Choosing a healthy snack, going for a short walk instead of skipping movement, or preparing a balanced meal at home are all examples of positive steps that deserve recognition.

Each time you follow through on a healthy choice, you reinforce your belief in your ability to make positive changes. These small wins help you see progress, even when the scale doesn't move right away. They also provide a steady source of motivation, reminding you that your efforts matter and are leading you in the right direction.

Confidence grows from these consistent actions. As you collect more small wins, you start to trust yourself and your new routines. Even setbacks feel less discouraging because you know you can get back on track. Confidence isn't something that happens overnight; it's built gradually by proving to yourself, over and over, that you are capable of making good decisions for your health.

Celebrate your small wins and let them fuel your confidence. Over time, these moments of success become the foundation for lasting change, helping you maintain your progress and continue reaching new goals.

CHAPTER 5

The Science of Nutrition

— ⋈ —

Nutrition is often made more complicated than it needs to be, with endless rules, trends, and conflicting advice. In reality, the fundamentals of healthy eating are straightforward and grounded in science, rather than marketing or quick-fix promises. Understanding the basics gives you the tools to make better choices without feeling overwhelmed or restricted.

In this chapter, you'll learn what really matters when it comes to food and how to nourish your body for steady energy, strength, and weight loss. We'll examine the roles of various nutrients, explore practical ways to balance your meals, and discuss strategies to enjoy food while supporting your goals. With straightforward guidance, you can feel confident about what you eat and focus on habits that make a real difference.

What really matters?

All foods are made up of three main macronutrients: carbohydrates, proteins, and fats. Each plays a unique role in your body and is essential for good health, especially during weight loss.

Carbohydrates are your body's primary source of energy. They're found in foods like fruits, vegetables, grains, and legumes. While some diets recommend eliminating carbs entirely, the key is to focus on high-quality sources, such as whole grains, beans, and fresh produce. These foods provide steady energy, fiber for digestion, and essential vitamins.

Proteins are the building blocks for your muscles, skin, hair, and other tissues. Eating enough protein helps you maintain muscle as you lose weight, keeps you feeling full longer, and supports your immune system. Good protein sources include lean meats, fish, eggs, beans, lentils, tofu, and dairy products.

Fats are often misunderstood, but they're just as important as the other macronutrients. Healthy fats help the body absorb vitamins, protect organs, and provide long-lasting energy. Focus on sources like avocados, nuts, seeds, olives, and oils, such as olive or canola oil.

Rather than cutting out any group, aim to include all three macronutrients in your meals. This balanced approach helps your body function well, keeps your hunger in check, and makes meals more satisfying. When you understand the basics of macronutrients, it becomes easier to build healthy meals and reach your weight loss goals in a way that feels sustainable.

Balancing meals for women

A balanced meal includes a mix of carbohydrates, protein, and healthy fats, along with plenty of fiber from fruits and vegetables. This combination helps maintain steady energy levels, supports your metabolism, and makes it easier to manage hunger and cravings throughout the day.

For women, balanced meals are essential because nutritional needs can shift with age, activity level, and hormonal changes. Starting with a source of lean protein, such as eggs, chicken, beans, or yogurt, helps preserve muscle and keeps you feeling satisfied for longer. Add a serving of complex carbohydrates, such as whole grains or starchy vegetables, to boost energy and fiber intake. Include healthy fats, like a drizzle of olive oil, a handful of nuts, or slices of avocado, to support hormone balance and help your body absorb vitamins.

Don't forget plenty of colorful vegetables and fruits. These foods are packed with nutrients and add volume to your meals without adding extra calories. They also provide the antioxidants and minerals your body needs for long-term health.

Balancing your plate doesn't have to be complicated. Try to make half your plate vegetables, one-quarter lean protein, and one-quarter whole grains or starchy vegetables. Add a small portion of healthy fats to round out the meal. This straightforward approach simplifies meal planning, supporting both weight loss and overall well-being.

The truth about calories

Calories are a measure of the energy your body gets from food and drinks. While they're often the focus of weight loss advice, calories alone don't tell the whole story. Understanding how they work can help you make better choices without feeling restricted or confused.

Your body requires a specific number of calories each day to perform basic functions, such as breathing, thinking, and moving. When you consume more calories than your body needs, the excess energy is stored as fat. Eating fewer calories than you burn over time leads to weight loss.

But not all calories are created equal. The source of your calories matters. A balanced meal with lean protein, whole grains, and plenty of vegetables will keep you satisfied and nourished far better than the same number of calories from processed snacks or sugary drinks. High-quality foods provide more vitamins, minerals, and fiber, which help you feel fuller and support your health in the long run.

It's also important not to cut calories too low. Eating too little can slow your metabolism, leave you feeling tired, and even cause muscle loss. Instead, aim for a gentle calorie deficit enough to see steady progress without feeling deprived.

Focusing on the quality of your food, listening to your body's hunger signals, and maintaining consistent, balanced meals will help you naturally manage your calories. When you approach calories with this mindset, healthy eating and weight loss become much more manageable and less stressful.

Hydration and its surprising effects

Staying well-hydrated is one of the simplest ways to support your health and weight loss goals, yet it's often overlooked. Water plays a crucial role in nearly every function of the body, from digestion and circulation to regulating body temperature and supporting clear thinking.

Drinking enough water can help control hunger and reduce the urge to snack, as thirst is sometimes mistaken for hunger. Starting your day with a glass of water and sipping it regularly throughout the day can help keep your energy steady and avoid unnecessary calories from sugary drinks or mindless snacking.

Proper hydration also helps your body burn fat more efficiently, flush out waste, and maintain healthy-looking skin. It's essential to drink more water when you're active, spending time in hot weather, or eating foods high in fiber.

Aim for approximately eight glasses a day, but note that your body's needs may vary depending on your activity level, age, and climate. Carrying a water bottle and keeping it in sight can serve as a helpful reminder.

Making hydration a daily habit is a small change that brings significant benefits for your energy, focus, and overall progress on your weight loss journey.

Understanding portion control

Portion control about knows how much food your body truly needs, rather than relying on large servings or eating until you're overly full. Even healthy foods can lead to weight gain if portions are too big, so learning to recognize the correct amount is key to steady progress.

Start by paying attention to your hunger and fullness cues. Eat slowly, and check in with yourself during meals. Are you satisfied, or just finishing what's on your plate out of habit? It's helpful to serve meals on smaller plates or bowls, which can naturally make portions more reasonable.

You can also use simple visual cues:

- A serving of protein (like chicken or fish) is about the size of your palm.
- One cup of cooked grains or pasta is roughly a fist.
- Healthy fats, like nuts or cheese, should be about the size of your thumb.

Restaurants and packaged foods often have much larger portions than you need, so don't feel pressured to clean your plate. Take leftovers home or ask for a half portion when dining out.

Practicing portion control doesn't mean you have to feel deprived. It's about enjoying your meals, paying attention to your body, and making choices that help you reach your goals one balanced plate at a time.

Whole foods vs. processed foods

Choosing what to eat is about more than just counting calories or grams of fat; it's also about the quality of your food. Whole foods are foods that are as close to their natural state as possible. These include fresh fruits and vegetables, whole grains, lean meats, fish, beans, nuts, and seeds. They provide your body with essential nutrients, fiber, and antioxidants that help keep you healthy, satisfied, and full of energy.

Processed foods, on the other hand, have been changed from their original form through manufacturing. They often contain added sugars, salt, unhealthy fats, preservatives, and artificial ingredients. Typical examples are packaged snacks, sugary drinks, instant noodles, white bread, and fast food.

While it's okay to enjoy processed foods occasionally, relying on them too much can make weight loss harder and affect your health over time. These foods are often high in calories but low in nutrients, making it easier to overeat without feeling full.

Your meals with mostly whole foods give you more control over what you're eating and support your long-term goals. It also helps you develop a better relationship with food, where meals are both nourishing and enjoyable. When you make whole foods the central part of your diet, you'll likely notice more energy, fewer cravings, and more steady progress on your journey.

Eating out without stress

Dining out is a part of life, whether it's meeting friends, family celebrations, or simply taking a break from cooking. With a few practical strategies, you can enjoy meals out without feeling anxious or losing sight of your health and wellness goals.

Start by looking at the menu ahead of time. This allows you to plan your choices and explore options with lean protein, vegetables, and whole grains. Don't be afraid to ask for substitutions, such as a side of salad instead of fries or grilled chicken instead of a fried option. Restaurants are accustomed to special requests, and most are happy to accommodate them.

Pay attention to portion sizes, as restaurant meals are often much larger than you need. Consider sharing a main dish, asking for a half-portion, or packing up leftovers to take home. Eat slowly, enjoy each bite, and listen to your body's cues for fullness.

Try to stick with water, unsweetened tea, or other low-calorie drinks instead of sugary sodas or cocktails. If you want dessert, consider asking someone to split it with you, so you can enjoy a treat without overindulging.

One meal out will not undo your progress. Focus on enjoying the experience and making the best choices you can in the moment. Over time, these small, mindful actions add up and help you build confidence in your ability to handle any eating situation with less stress.

CHAPTER 6

Empowered Eating & Mindfulness

———————— ·✕· ————————

Eating well is about more than following rules or sticking to a strict plan. Empowered eating means making choices that honor your body's needs, preferences, and hunger signals, all while enjoying your meals without guilt. Mindfulness helps you slow down, pay attention to how food affects your body, and break free from old habits that no longer serve you.

In this chapter, you'll discover how to tune in to your body's signals, build a positive relationship with food, and develop new routines that make healthy eating feel natural and enjoyable. Empowered, mindful eating is not about perfection; it's about awareness, flexibility, and trust in yourself.

What empowered eating is (and isn't)

Empowered eating is about making food choices from a place of self-respect and awareness, not from guilt or pressure. It means listening to your body's signals for hunger and fullness, choosing foods that make you feel good, and allowing yourself to enjoy eating without judgment or strict rules.

Empowered eating is not about perfection or following the latest trend. It isn't about depriving yourself or labeling foods as "good" or "bad." Instead, it encourages you to focus on how different foods affect your energy, mood, and well-being. When you eat mindfully and with intention, you learn to trust your body and respond to its needs rather than external diet rules.

It's also about flexibility. Life brings special occasions, cravings, and busy days. Empowered eating allows for these moments without guilt, knowing that one meal or treat doesn't define your health or progress. Over time, this approach helps you build a balanced relationship with food, one where eating supports both your goals and your enjoyment of life.

Mindful eating practices for daily life

Mindful eating is about paying full attention to your food, your body, and your eating experience. By slowing down and tuning in, you become more aware of what you eat and how it affects your body. This simple shift can help you enjoy meals more, recognize true hunger and fullness, and avoid overeating.

Here are some practical ways to bring mindfulness into your daily meals:

- **Pause before you eat.** Take a moment to notice your hunger level and mood before starting a meal or snack.

- **Minimize distractions.** Turn off screens and try to eat at a table, focusing on your food and the people you're with.
- **Eat slowly.** Put your fork down between bites, chew thoroughly, and savor each flavor and texture.
- **Notice your senses.** Appreciate the colors, smells, and presentation of your food. This can help increase satisfaction and enjoyment.
- **Check in with your body.** Halfway through your meal, pause and ask yourself if you're still hungry or starting to feel satisfied.
- **Respect fullness.** Stop eating when you feel comfortably full, even if there's food left on your plate.

Practicing mindful eating takes time, but even small changes can help you build a healthier relationship with food. The more you listen to your body and focus on the experience of eating, the easier it becomes to make choices that truly support your well-being.

Ending the "all-or-nothing" mentality

Many women fall into the trap of thinking that healthy eating is all or nothing; you're either completely "on track" or you've failed. This rigid mindset can make even small slips feel like major setbacks, leading to feelings of guilt, frustration, or even giving up entirely. In reality, lasting change comes from flexibility, not perfection.

Letting go of the all-or-nothing mentality starts with accepting that no one eats perfectly all the time. Life is full of special occasions, busy days, and moments of stress. Instead of aiming for flawless habits, focus on making the best choices you can in each situation. If you have a treat or a bigger meal than planned, see it as a regular part of life, not a reason to give up on your goals.

Every healthy choice counts, even if it's just one good decision in a challenging day. Over time, these small efforts add up and help you build confidence in your ability to stay on track. When you're gentle with yourself and flexible in your approach, you're much more likely to enjoy your journey and keep making progress, no matter what comes your way.

Managing cravings without shame

Cravings are a regular part of life, not a sign of weakness or failure. Many women feel embarrassed or frustrated when they crave certain foods, especially if those foods don't fit their idea of a "perfect" diet. But shaming yourself for having cravings only makes them harder to handle and can lead to cycles of restriction and overeating.

The first step is to accept cravings as a natural response sometimes triggered by emotions, stress, hormonal changes, or simply seeing or smelling food you enjoy. Rather than fighting the urge or judging yourself, pause and notice what you're feeling. Are you truly hungry, or is something else at play, like boredom or stress?

If you're physically hungry, it's okay to satisfy your craving reasonably. Enjoy a small portion of the food you want, eat it slowly, and pay attention to the taste and how you feel. Often, this mindful approach helps you feel satisfied with less.

If the craving isn't about hunger, try to meet your needs in a different way, such as going for a walk, drinking a glass of water, or calling a friend. The goal is to respond to cravings with curiosity and care, not guilt or harsh rules.

Managing cravings without shame enables you to make better choices and cultivate a healthier relationship with food, one where enjoying what you eat becomes a source of comfort and joy, rather than stress or regret.

Navigating social and family pressure

Making healthy choices can feel more challenging when friends, family, or colleagues don't share your goals or habits. Social situations often involve food, and well-meaning loved ones may encourage you to eat more, try treats, or skip your usual routines. These moments can create pressure to abandon your plans or leave you feeling awkward about saying no.

The key is to approach these situations with confidence and kindness. You don't need to explain your choices in detail or feel guilty for putting your health first. A simple, polite response, such as "I'm good for now, thank you" or "That looks great, but I'm full," is usually enough. Most people will respect your decision, especially if you stay consistent.

It also helps to plan. If you know you'll be at a gathering with tempting foods, consider having a healthy snack beforehand, offer to bring a dish you enjoy, or scan the menu for options that fit your dietary needs. Surround yourself with people who support your efforts, and remember that one meal or event won't undo your progress.

If you do choose to indulge, enjoy it without guilt. Healthy living is about balance, not perfection. Over time, your confidence in managing social and family pressure will grow, making it easier to stay true to your goals no matter what's on the table.

Intuitive eating: listening to your body

Intuitive eating about trusts your body to guide your food choices, rather than following strict diets or outside rules. It means paying attention to your hunger and fullness signals, choosing foods that satisfy and nourish you, and letting go of guilt or judgment around eating.

Begin by checking in with yourself before meals and snacks. Are you truly hungry, or are you eating out of habit, boredom, or emotion? Learn to recognize what real hunger feels like, typically characterized by a gentle emptiness or a growling sensation in your stomach. When you eat, focus on how each bite tastes and how your body responds. Slow down, and stop when you feel comfortably satisfied, not stuffed.

Intuitive eating also means mindfully honoring your cravings. If you want something sweet or savory, allow yourself a small portion, savor it, and notice how it makes you feel. You'll often find that satisfaction comes from truly enjoying your food, not from overeating.

Listening to your body helps you develop a healthier, more balanced relationship with food. You learn to trust your instincts, make choices that feel good, and support your well-being without stress or rigid rules. This approach turns eating into a positive, nourishing experience that fits your real life.

CHAPTER 7

Decoding Diets & Trends

Every year brings a new wave of diets and nutrition trends, each promising quick results and a simple path to weight loss. It's easy to feel overwhelmed or confused by all the advice, especially when different plans offer conflicting information. In reality, there is no one-size-fits-all solution, and what works for someone else may not work for you.

This chapter takes a closer look at popular diets and trends, exploring what's helpful, what's hype, and how to sort fact from fiction. By understanding the pros and cons of different approaches, you can make informed choices and create an eating plan that genuinely supports your health and fits your lifestyle.

A critical look at popular diets

Popular diets often make headlines with promises of fast results and dramatic changes. From low-carb and keto to intermittent fasting and plant-based plans, each approach has its champions and critics. While some people achieve short-term success, it's essential to understand both the benefits and limitations of any specific diet before committing to it.

Many popular diets work at first because they create structure, limit certain foods, or reduce overall calorie intake. However, strict rules can sometimes lead to feelings of deprivation, making it harder to maintain the plan over time. Diets that eliminate whole food groups may also make it challenging to get all the nutrients your body needs.

Some approaches, such as Mediterranean or balanced plant-based diets, are supported by substantial research and focus on whole foods, healthy fats, and an abundance of fruits and vegetables. Others, such as extreme low-calorie or highly restrictive plans, may bring quick results but can be challenging to sustain and may even harm your health in the long run.

It's also important to watch for diet trends driven more by marketing than by science. Be cautious of plans that rely heavily on supplements, packaged meals, or "detox" products. These often promise more than they deliver and can be expensive, yet fail to offer lasting results.

The most effective diet is one you can follow comfortably for the long term, one that fits your lifestyle, supports your health, and allows for flexibility. Taking a critical look at popular diets helps you avoid common pitfalls and find an approach that works for you, rather than chasing every new trend.

Why "best diet" is personal

The idea that there is a single "best diet" for everyone is a myth. Each person's body, preferences, lifestyle, and health needs are different. What works well for one person may not fit another's daily routine, food culture, or nutritional requirements.

Your unique genetics, metabolism, medical history, and even your schedule all play a role in how your body responds to certain foods and meal patterns. Some people feel their best eating mostly plant-based meals, while others need more protein or do better with frequent, smaller meals throughout the day. Food intolerances, allergies, and personal tastes matter, too.

Sustainability is also a key factor. The best diet is one you can enjoy and maintain over time, not just for a few weeks. If a plan feels too restrictive or doesn't fit your family life, you're less likely to stick with it. Flexibility, enjoyment, and satisfaction are just as important as nutrition when choosing an eating approach.

The proper diet for you is the one that meets your body's needs, supports your health, and fits naturally into your life. By focusing on what makes you feel good and what you can realistically sustain, you're far more likely to reach your goals and maintain your progress for the long term.

Breaking up with fad diets

Fad diets often promise rapid weight loss and a fresh start, but they rarely lead to lasting results. These plans are usually built on strict rules, extreme restrictions, or the elimination of entire food groups. While the excitement of quick progress can be tempting, the reality is that most fad diets are hard to follow for more than a short time.

Following these plans can leave you feeling deprived, isolated, or frustrated, especially when social events or busy days make it challenging to stick to the rules. Worse, the cycle of starting and stopping fad diets can lead to weight regain and damage your relationship with food. You might end up feeling discouraged or convinced that you "lack willpower," when the real problem is the diet itself.

Breaking up with fad diets means shifting your focus from temporary fixes to long-term habits. Select an approach that enables you to enjoy a diverse range of foods, accommodates your preferences, and suits your daily routine. Pay attention to how foods make you feel and look for balance, not perfection.

Letting go of fad diets frees you to build a healthier relationship with eating — one based on trust, flexibility, and real nourishment. Over time, this approach fosters greater confidence, reduced stress, and more lasting results.

The evidence behind sustainable eating

Years of research have shown that the most effective approach to achieving weight loss and improved health is not a quick-fix diet, but a pattern of eating that you can maintain over time. Sustainable eating means focusing on habits that are flexible, enjoyable, and supportive of your overall well-being, not just your waistline.

Studies consistently find that people are more likely to reach and maintain a healthy weight when they choose mostly whole, minimally processed foods, eat regular meals, and include a wide variety of nutrients. Diets rich in vegetables, fruits, whole grains, lean proteins, and healthy fats are associated with lower rates of chronic disease, improved energy levels, and greater satisfaction with eating.

Sustainable eating also allows for occasional treats and social occasions, making it possible to maintain healthy habits in the long term. Instead of relying on willpower alone, you develop practical strategies that work in real life, like planning meals, enjoying favorite foods in moderation, and listening to your body's natural hunger cues.

Focusing on sustainable habits rather than temporary fixes, you're more likely to see steady progress, feel better day-to-day, and avoid the cycle of yo-yo dieting. The evidence is clear: when healthy eating aligns with your lifestyle, it becomes easier to maintain, more enjoyable, and ultimately more successful in the long run.

How to make your own nutrition rules

Creating your own nutrition rules gives you the freedom to build healthy habits that truly fit your life. Instead of following someone else's plan, you choose guidelines that reflect your needs, preferences, and goals. This approach makes eating feel less restrictive and more sustainable.

Begin by paying attention to how different foods affect you physically and emotionally. Notice which meals leave you satisfied and energized, and which ones tend to cause cravings or sluggishness. Use this information to shape your everyday choices.

Keep your rules flexible and straightforward. For example, you might eat vegetables with most meals, include a source of protein at breakfast, or keep sugary drinks as an occasional treat. Some people find it helpful to follow the "80/20 rule" eating well most of the time, while allowing room for favorite foods in moderation.

Personalize your guidelines to match your routine. If you're busy during the week, plan easy-to-prep meals or healthy snacks you can grab on the go. If you enjoy eating out, consider setting a rule to check menus ahead of time or splitting larger portions.

These rules are meant to support your well-being, not to create more stress. Review them regularly and adjust as your needs change. By making your own nutrition rules, you build confidence, maintain balance, and develop a way of eating that you can enjoy for years to come.

Transitioning to healthier habits

Shifting to healthier habits doesn't have to be overwhelming or happen all at once. Lasting change often comes from small, steady steps that build over time. Begin by choosing one or two simple changes that feel manageable, such as adding an extra serving of vegetables to your daily diet, drinking more water, or cooking at home more often.

Focus on progress, not perfection. Some days will go smoothly, while others may bring setbacks or old habits. That's normal. Celebrate each positive choice, no matter how small, and use any challenges as opportunities to learn what works best for you.

It can be helpful to set reminders or track your new habits in a journal or a dedicated app. This keeps you motivated and lets you see how far you've come. Involve friends or family for support, or find an accountability partner to share your goals and celebrate your successes.

Be patient with yourself during this transition. Real change takes time, and healthy habits become easier with practice. As these new routines start to feel natural, you'll notice improvements in your energy, mood, and confidence, and your progress will be much easier to maintain in the long run.

CHAPTER 8

Physical Activity, More Than Just Exercise

— ⋈ —

Moving your body is about much more than burning calories or reaching a certain weight. Physical activity is key to overall health, energy, and well-being. It can boost your mood, support your metabolism, and help you manage stress, all while building strength and confidence in your daily life.

This chapter explores various ways to stay active, from structured workouts to simple movements that can be incorporated into your routine. You'll learn how to find activities you enjoy, overcome common obstacles, and make movement a regular, rewarding part of your lifestyle. Whether you're new to exercise or looking to try something different, you'll find practical tips to help you stay motivated and active in a way that works for you.

The role of movement in women's health

Movement plays a vital role in women's health, offering benefits that reach far beyond weight loss. Regular physical activity helps support heart health, strengthens bones, and maintains healthy muscles and joints. It also boosts your mood, lowers stress, and improves sleep, factors that are especially important for women at every stage of life.

Exercise can help regulate hormone levels, which may alleviate symptoms associated with the menstrual cycle, pregnancy, or menopause. Staying active is also linked to a reduced risk of chronic diseases such as diabetes, high blood pressure, and certain types of cancer.

You don't need to spend hours at the gym to see these benefits. Even moderate activities, such as brisk walking, gardening, or dancing, can make a significant difference. The key is to find forms of movement you enjoy and to make them a regular part of your routine.

By prioritizing your health, you not only support your physical well-being but also build confidence and resilience. The positive effects carry over into all areas of your life, helping you feel stronger, more capable, and better equipped to handle daily challenges.

Finding exercise you actually enjoy

Sticking to an exercise routine is much easier when you genuinely enjoy what you're doing. The idea that you must spend hours at the gym or follow a strict plan isn't accurate for everyone. What matters most is discovering types of movement that feel good and fit naturally into your life.

Start by exploring different activities: walk in your neighborhood, try a dance or yoga class, swim, cycle, or experiment with home work out videos. Notice which options leave you feeling energized or uplifted. If you're unsure where to start, think back to activities you enjoyed as a child or consider joining a group class for a sense of community and fun.

Listen to your body and your mood. Some days you might want something high-energy, like a group fitness class, while other times a peaceful walk or gentle stretching is what you need. Mixing up your routine keeps things interesting and helps you work different muscle groups.

Invite a friend or family member to join you for added motivation and accountability. Remember, there's no "right" way to exercise; what's most important is that you keep moving in ways you find rewarding. When you enjoy your workouts, staying active feels less like a chore and more like a natural, positive part of your life.

Home vs. gym workouts

Both home and gym workouts offer unique benefits, and the best choice depends on your preferences, schedule, and resources. Understanding the differences can help you create a routine that feels manageable and enjoyable.

Home workouts offer convenience and flexibility. You can exercise anytime, save travel time, and often need little or no equipment. Home routines are great for busy schedules or those who prefer privacy. Online classes, workout apps, and simple routines, such as bodyweight exercises or yoga, make it easy to stay active at home.

Gym workouts provide access to a broader range of equipment, classes, and sometimes professional guidance. Gyms can offer motivation through group energy, a social environment, and the structure of scheduled classes. They're ideal for people who enjoy variety, want access to weights and machines, or benefit from a community atmosphere.

Here's a comparison to help you decide:

No travel needed	Access to more equipment and classes
Flexible scheduling	Professional support and trainers
Private, comfortable environment	Motivating group atmosphere
Minimal or no equipment required	Wide variety of workout options
Cost-effective	Additional cost for membership
Ideal for short sessions or busy days	Great for structured, longer workouts

Some people enjoy mixing both options, using the gym for strength training or classes, and home for quick routines or stretching. The key is to choose what fits your life, helps you stay consistent, and keeps you motivated to move. No matter where you exercise, the benefits are real, so pick the environment that helps you thrive.

Movement for every fitness level

Regardless of your starting point, there is a way to move your body that suits your needs and abilities. Physical activity doesn't have to mean intense workouts or long gym sessions. The most crucial step is to find a level of movement that feels safe, comfortable, and motivating for you.

If you're new to exercise or coming back after a break, start with gentle activities like walking, stretching, or beginner yoga. Even a few minutes a day can help you build strength and confidence. For those with more experience, adding resistance training, cycling, or group classes can provide new challenges and keep things interesting.

It's helpful to listen to your body and adjust your routine as needed. Some days will call for a slower pace or lighter activity, while others may require more vigorous activity. Focus on progress, not perfection, and celebrate each step forward.

Here are examples of movements for different fitness levels:

Gentle walking	Brisk walking/jogging	Running/intervals
Chair exercises	Bodyweight strength	Weighted strength
Light stretching	Pilates/yoga	Power yoga
Wall push-ups	Modified push-ups	Full push-ups
Step-ups on stairs	Aerobic dance	HIIT workouts

Remember, everyone starts somewhere. Choose activities you enjoy and go at your own pace. Over time, your endurance and strength will improve, making it easier to try new things and stay active for the long term.

Benefits of strength training

Strength training is an integral part of any well-rounded fitness routine, and its benefits go far beyond building muscle. For women, incorporating regular strength exercises can help boost metabolism, support healthy bones, and enhance body composition by reducing body fat and increasing lean muscle mass.

Strength training also helps maintain and build bone density, which is especially important as women age and the risk of osteoporosis rises. It supports better balance and coordination, reducing the risk of falls and injuries in daily life.

Beyond the physical advantages, strength training can boost your confidence and mental well-being. It provides a sense of accomplishment as you notice progress, whether you're lifting heavier weights, doing more repetitions, or simply feeling stronger in everyday activities.

Regular strength training can help regulate blood sugar, support heart health, and make it easier to manage your weight by increasing the calories you burn even at rest. With options ranging from bodyweight moves at home to free weights at the gym, there are routines to fit every level.

Including strength training in your weekly routine supports your health now and in the future, making daily tasks easier and giving you the strength to stay active for life.

Cardio, flexibility, and mobility basics

A balanced approach to movement includes more than just strength exercises. Cardio, flexibility, and mobility are all essential for overall health and well-being.

Cardio (aerobic exercise) involves activities that raise your heart rate and increase blood flow. Walking, cycling, swimming, and dancing are all forms of cardio. These activities strengthen your heart and lungs, improve endurance, help with weight management, and boost your mood by releasing feel-good hormones.

Flexibility is your body's ability to move joints and muscles through a full range of motion. Gentle stretching, yoga, and Pilates can improve flexibility, which helps prevent injuries, ease muscle stiffness, and make daily movements more comfortable.

Mobility focuses on how well you can move your body, especially at your joints. Mobility exercises, such as arm circles, hip openers, and ankle rolls, support better posture, balance, and coordination. Improved mobility can also make your workouts safer and more effective.

Combining cardio, flexibility, and mobility exercises with strength training creates a complete routine. This well-rounded approach keeps your body strong, balanced, and able to handle the demands of everyday life. Even a few minutes a day devoted to each area can bring noticeable benefits over time.

Building your personal activity plan

Creating a personal activity plan helps you stay consistent and motivated, making it easier to incorporate movement into your daily life. The best plan is one that aligns with your goals, preferences, schedule, and fitness level, while also allowing for flexibility as life changes.

Begin by considering your primary objectives. Are you hoping to boost energy, lose weight, build strength, or reduce stress? Your goals will help you decide which activities to focus on most. For example, to improve heart health, incorporate more cardio; to build strength, add strength training.

Next, review your weekly schedule and identify pockets of time for activities. Even short sessions, such as a 10-minute walk after meals or a quick stretching routine before bed, add up over the week. Choose a mix of activities you enjoy, such as walking, cycling, yoga, or home workouts, and try to include a combination of cardio, strength, and flexibility exercises.

It may help to write out your plan. Here's a simple example:

Monday	20-minute walk + stretching
Tuesday	Strength training at home
Wednesday	Yoga or gentle stretching
Thursday	Cardio (cycling or dancing)
Friday	Bodyweight circuit
Saturday	Rest or light activity
Sunday	Family hike or outdoor walk

Listen to your body and make changes as needed. If you miss a session, simply pick up where you left off. Celebrate your progress, adjust your plan as your interests and abilities grow, and remember: the most effective activity plan is the one you can stick with and enjoy.

Preventing injury and burnout

Staying active is essential, but pushing too hard or skipping recovery can lead to injuries and burnout? Taking care of your body ensures you can continue to move and enjoy exercise in the long term.

Start by warming up before each workout with gentle movements or light cardio. Warming up prepares your muscles and joints, helping prevent strains and sprains. Likewise, cooling down with stretching or slow movements gives your body time to recover and reduces soreness. Listen to your body's signals if you feel pain beyond normal muscle fatigue, pause, and assess whether you need to rest or adjust your routine. Don't ignore aches, sharp pains, or swelling, as these may be signs you need a break or to seek medical advice.

Rest days are just as important as active days. Allow your muscles time to recover and rebuild by incorporating one or two rest days into your weekly routine. Mix up your routine with different activities to avoid overusing the same muscles and keep things interesting.

Stay hydrated and eats nourishing foods to support recovery. If you feel mentally drained or lose motivation, consider switching to a different activity, lowering the intensity, or taking a short break to refresh your outlook.

Balancing effort with recovery can help reduce your risk of injury and prevent burnout. This approach helps you stay consistent and make movement a positive, sustainable part of your lifestyle.

CHAPTER 9

Metabolism & Plateaus

—————— ·✕· ——————

Metabolism is often a buzzword in weight loss discussions, yet it's commonly misunderstood. While a healthy metabolism plays a significant role in how your body uses energy, many factors can influence how quickly or slowly you see results. Hitting a plateau, where progress seems to stall despite your efforts, is also a regular part of many health journeys.

This chapter explains how metabolism works, why plateaus happen, and what you can do to support steady progress. By understanding these key concepts, you'll be better equipped to adjust your habits, break through slow periods, and stay motivated for the long run.

What "boosting metabolism" really means

"Boosting metabolism" is a phrase frequently used in weight loss conversations, but it's crucial to understand what it truly entails. Metabolism is the process your body uses to turn food into energy. It works around the clock, powering everything from breathing and digestion to movement and thinking.

While some people have naturally faster or slower metabolisms due to genetics, age, or body composition, there are healthy ways to support and optimize this process. Building muscle through regular strength training is one of the most effective methods, since muscle tissue burns more calories than fat, even at rest. Staying active throughout the day by walking, taking the stairs, or simply moving more also keeps your metabolism engaged.

Eating regular, balanced meals helps prevent your body from entering "conservation mode," which can occur when you skip meals or drastically reduce your calorie intake. Drinking enough water and getting enough sleep further support healthy metabolic function.

It's important to remember that there are no magic solutions or shortcuts. Most products or supplements claiming to "speed up" metabolism offer little real benefit. The most effective way to support your metabolism is through a combination of consistent movement, balanced nutrition, and healthy daily habits. These changes not only aid in weight loss but also enhance your overall energy and well-being.

Natural ways to increase metabolism

Supporting your metabolism doesn't require extreme measures or special products. Several simple, natural strategies can help your body use energy more efficiently and support your weight loss efforts.

1. Build muscle with strength training:

Muscle burns more calories than fat, even when you're at rest. Incorporating strength exercises, such as squats, push-ups, or weightlifting, just a few times a week can gradually increase your resting metabolic rate.

2. Stay active throughout the day:

Regular movement keeps your metabolism engaged. Look for opportunities to add activity, such as taking the stairs, walking during breaks, or standing while on the phone.

3. Eat enough protein:

Protein-rich foods not only help build and maintain muscle, but also require more energy to digest compared to fats or carbohydrates. Including a source of protein at each meal supports your metabolism and helps you feel full longer.

4. Don't skip meals:

Eating regular, balanced meals helps keep your metabolism steady. Skipping meals or drastically cutting calories can slow down your metabolic rate and make it harder to lose weight.

5. Stay hydrated:

Water is essential for all your body's processes, including metabolism. Drinking enough fluids each day helps your body burn calories more efficiently.

6. Get enough sleep:

Poor sleep can disrupt the hormones that control hunger and metabolism. Aim for 7–9 hours of restful sleep each night to support your body's natural rhythms.

These natural habits work together to help your metabolism function optimally. Focus on incorporating them into your routine, and you'll support not just weight loss, but also your overall health and energy.

The effects of age, hormones, and menopause

As women age, natural changes in the body can influence metabolism, energy levels, and weight gain or loss. Hormones play a central role in these shifts, especially during key life stages such as per menopause and menopause.

During the years leading up to menopause, levels of estrogen and other hormones begin to fluctuate. These changes can affect how your body stores fat, often making it easier to gain weight, especially around the midsection, even if you're eating and activity habits stay the same. Metabolism also tends to slow down with age, partly due to the gradual loss of muscle mass and changes in physical activity.

Sleep disruptions, mood changes, and increased stress are also common during this period, and all can impact weight management. It's normal to find that what worked in your twenties or thirties may need adjustment as you move through your forties and beyond.

The good news is that healthy habits remain powerful tools at every stage of life. Staying active, focusing on strength training to support muscle, eating balanced meals, and prioritizing quality sleep can help manage these changes. If you're experiencing symptoms that impact your daily life or weight management, it may be beneficial to consult with your healthcare provider for personalized guidance.

Understanding the effects of age, hormones, and menopause allows you to approach these transitions with patience and realistic expectations. By adapting your routine to your body's current needs, you can support your health, well-being, and progress at every stage of life.

Overcoming plateaus with science

Hitting a plateau where progress stalls even though you're following your plan is a regular part of many weight loss journeys. It may not be very encouraging, but understanding why plateaus occur and utilizing proven strategies can help you move forward.

Plateaus occur because your body adapts to new routines. As you lose weight, your metabolism may slow down slightly, and you may burn fewer calories during daily activities. Sometimes, habits like mindless snacking or reduced physical activity can creep in without you noticing.

To overcome a plateau, start by reviewing your daily habits. Keeping a simple food and activity journal can help you spot patterns or areas for improvement. Small changes, such as adjusting portion sizes or incorporating a new type of exercise, can jump-start progress again.

Science shows that mixing up your workouts by increasing intensity, trying new activities, or incorporating strength training can challenge your body and boost results. Focusing on non-scale victories, like improved energy or fitness, helps you stay motivated while your body adjusts.

It's also important to be patient. Plateaus are often temporary, and sometimes your body needs time to reset. Stay consistent with your healthy habits, and remember that slow, steady progress leads to better results that last.

If a plateau persists, consider consulting a registered dietitian or healthcare professional for personalized guidance. With the right strategies and mindset, you can break through plateaus and continue moving toward your goals.

Adjusting habits for long-term results

Sticking with the same routine for too long can sometimes lead to stalled progress or loss of motivation. That's why it's essential to check in with your habits from time to time and make minor adjustments as your needs and goals change. This approach helps you stay engaged, overcome plateaus, and build a healthier lifestyle that truly lasts.

Start by taking a closer look at your daily choices. Are old habits creeping back, such as extra snacking or skipping workouts? Your schedule has changed, and your old routine no longer fits as well. Adjusting doesn't mean starting over; it simply means making thoughtful tweaks that keep things fresh and realistic.

Try swapping out certain foods for healthier options, exploring new recipes, or adding a new activity you've never tried before. If you've been doing the same workout for months, challenge your body differently, take a new class, try interval training, or add more strength work.

It's also helpful to reset your goals as you progress. Celebrate the milestones you've reached and set new, realistic targets to keep yourself motivated. Remember, the best habits are those that fit your life and can adapt as it changes.

By being open to change and willing to adjust, you make it much easier to keep moving forward. This flexible mindset helps you maintain your results, avoid burnout, and feel good about your progress, no matter where you are on your journey.

Non-scale victories and how to track them

The number on the scale doesn't always measure progress. Some of the most meaningful changes happen in ways a scale can't show. These are known as non-scale victories, small and big improvements that reflect your hard work and healthier habits.

Non-scale victories include noticing your clothes fit better, having more energy during the day, or feeling stronger during workouts. Maybe you're sleeping more soundly, keeping up with your kids more easily, or managing stress in healthier ways. Positive changes in your mood, self-confidence, and relationship with food are also vital signs of progress.

To track these victories, keep a simple journal where you record weekly or monthly changes. Write down things like improved stamina, new healthy recipes you've tried, or compliments from friends and family. You might also take occasional progress photos, note how your favorite jeans fit, or keep track of personal bests in your workouts.

Celebrating non-scale victories helps you stay motivated, especially during times when the scale doesn't budge. These milestones remind you that every healthy choice matters and that you're making real, lasting progress inside and out. Over time, these wins add up, helping you build confidence and stay committed to your journey.

CHAPTER 10

Staying Empowered, Body, Mind, and Community

———————— ∙✗∙ ————————

True wellness extends beyond numbers on a scale or the frequency of your workouts. It's about feeling strong in your body, confident in your mind, and supported by those around you. Staying empowered on your health journey means building habits and routines that nourish every part of who you are.

In this chapter, you'll explore ways to maintain motivation, tap into the power of community, and nurture a positive mindset. You'll find practical strategies to help you celebrate your progress, stay connected to your goals, and inspire others along the way. When body, mind, and community work together, lasting change becomes both possible and enjoyable.

Building resilience and self-belief

Resilience is your ability to bounce back from setbacks and keep moving forward, even when things get tough. Self-belief is the quiet confidence that you can handle challenges and reach your goals. Together, these qualities are potent tools for lasting success in both weight loss and life.

Building resilience starts with how you talk to yourself. Instead of focusing on mistakes or missed days, remind yourself of your progress and the effort you're putting in. When obstacles arise, take a step back, breathe, and look for solutions rather than giving in to frustration.

Self-belief grows as you collect small wins and see the results of your hard work. Each healthy meal, completed workout, or moment of self-care adds to your sense of accomplishment. Over time, these positive choices become evidence that you're capable of more than you might have thought.

It's also helpful to surround yourself with encouragement. Spend time with people who believe in your potential, and don't hesitate to ask for support when you need it. Celebrate your victories, no matter how small, and use them as reminders that setbacks are just temporary, not a reflection of your worth.

Nurturing resilience and self-confidence, you give yourself the strength to persevere. These qualities enable you to face challenges with a positive outlook, stay committed to your goals, and savor the journey as you grow and change.

The importance of community and support

Reaching your health goals is much easier when you have a network of support. A community, whether it's friends, family, or a group with shared goals, can offer motivation, accountability, and practical help when you need it most.

Supportive relationships encourage us on tough days and are a way to celebrate victories, big or small. Sharing your journey with others helps you feel understood and less alone. Sometimes, just knowing someone is cheering you on can make all the difference in sticking with your plans.

You don't have to do everything on your own. Joining a walking group, attending fitness classes, or connecting with people online can help you find the community that fits your needs. These connections can also bring new ideas, tips, and a sense of belonging to your journey.

When you seek support and surround yourself with positive influences, you strengthen your commitment and confidence. Community isn't just about reaching your own goals; it's about building each other up and creating a foundation for lasting, shared success.

Using accountability for real progress

Accountability means having a way to check in on your goals and actions, either with you or with others. It can be a powerful motivator, helping you stay focused and honest as you move forward. Knowing that someone is cheering you on, or that you'll be reviewing your progress, encourages you to keep your promises even on the days when motivation runs low.

There are many ways to build accountability into your routine. You might share your goals with a friend, join a support group, or use a tracking app to log your meals and workouts. Some people find it helpful to set up regular check-ins, such as weekly calls, messages, or even brief notes to themselves about what's working and what needs adjusting.

The key is to choose a method that fits your lifestyle and makes you feel encouraged, not pressured. When accountability is positive and supportive, it helps you celebrate progress, learn from setbacks, and keep moving in the right direction. Over time, this steady focus on your goals becomes a habit, making real, lasting change much more achievable.

Celebrating your unique journey

Every health and wellness journey is different, and it's essential to recognize that your path is uniquely yours. Comparing yourself to others can be discouraging, so focus on the progress you've made, the habits you've built, and the personal milestones you've achieved.

Celebrating your journey doesn't have to involve grand gestures. Small acknowledgments, such as noting a week of consistent workouts, preparing a healthy meal you're proud of, or feeling more energized, can reinforce your confidence and motivation. These moments remind you that change is happening, even if it's not always reflected on the scale.

Take time to reflect on how far you've come and honor the effort you put in daily. Recognize both your achievements and the lessons learned along the way. By valuing your unique journey, you cultivate self-respect, stay motivated, and create a positive mindset that supports lasting, healthy change.

Setting new goals as you grow

Progress does not end when you hit your first target. That's often just the beginning of something even more meaningful. As your body, mindset, and lifestyle evolve, your goals should evolve with them. Setting new goals along the way keeps you engaged, motivated, and aware of how much you've grown inside and out.

Your first goal was weight-related or centered on fitting into a specific outfit. However, over time, you may find yourself prioritizing energy, sleep quality, mental clarity, or emotional resilience. This shift is natural. What matters most is that your goals continue to reflect your current values and the person you are becoming.

New goals don't have to be big or dramatic. The most powerful ones are often small and deeply personal. For example, you might aim to walk three days a week without needing reminders. Or maybe you want to try one new healthy recipe each week, spend 10 minutes journaling each night, or start lifting heavier weights. These may seem like small wins, but over time, they contribute to lasting change.

One of the best ways to set practical goals is to ask yourself questions like: *"What matters to me now?"*, *"What do I want to feel more of?"*, or *"What have I already proven I can do and what's next?"* These questions keep your goals aligned with your real life, rather than chasing ideas of success that may no longer serve you.

And remember, your goals can also be flexible, as life changes. You change. It's okay to revise your goals if they no longer feel right. That's not giving up, it's growing wiser. It's being honest about what you need today, not just what you thought you needed months ago.

Please keep a record of your goals as they change. Write them down, say them out loud, and check in regularly. Celebrate each time you move one step closer. Let each achievement permit you to dream a little bigger or shift directions entirely. You're not starting over, you're building on a foundation of experience, self-trust, and strength.

This is your journey. Keep setting goals that remind you of your potential and reflect the life you're creating, one mindful, empowered step at a time.

Giving back and inspiring others

As you evolve in your wellness journey, something powerful begins to happen: you realize that your transformation is not just about you. It's about the ripple effect you create. Every healthy choice, every act of self-love, every moment you choose to get back up after falling becomes an invitation for someone else to believe in themselves, too. And that is a giving back that goes far beyond the legacy of charity.

Giving back doesn't always require a grand gesture. It might start with sharing your story honestly, talking to a friend who feels stuck, or simply being a quiet example of consistency and grace. The way you live becomes a light.

You might volunteer in a local community class, mentor someone just starting their health journey, or even inspire your children by showing them what strength and self-care look like. These moments matter more than you know.

Inspiring others doesn't require perfection; it only asks for authenticity. When you share your setbacks and wins, others feel seen. When you say, "I've been there, and here's what helped me," you offer more hope than any textbook advice ever could. Your vulnerability becomes a bridge for connection. And through that connection, you build a sense of purpose that fuels you even when motivation fades.

Giving back is also a form of healing. As you support others, you reinforce your strength. You remember where you started. You honor how far you've come. You show up not because you have all the answers, but because you know what it's like to search for them.

Whether it's creating a wellness group, posting your weekly wins on social media, or just choosing kindness in everyday moments, your life becomes a quiet revolution. You don't need a spotlight to make a difference. Sometimes the most powerful impact comes from those who lead gently and live intentionally.

As you move forward, ask yourself: how can I use what I've learned to uplift someone else? Maybe it's just one person. Perhaps it's your whole circle. But know this, your journey matters, not just to you, but to the lives you'll touch simply by continuing to show up. That is the valid reward of growth: becoming the reason someone else believes they can grow, too.

CHAPTER 11
Troubleshooting & Special Challenges

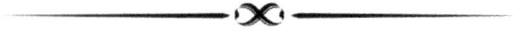

Even with the best intentions, most journeys come with unexpected detours. Weight loss and wellness are no different. There will be weeks when progress slows, moments when motivation fades, and times when life throws something your way that makes it hard to stay on track. That's not failure, it's real life.

This chapter is here to support you through those moments. Whether you're facing a plateau, dealing with health conditions, managing a busy family life, or just feeling emotionally drained, there are practical ways to respond without giving up or falling into old patterns.

Here, you'll find clear, compassionate guidance for navigating special situations and roadblocks that many women face. From emotional eating relapses to dealing with travel or illness, this chapter equips you with realistic tools to adapt, reset, and keep going with clarity and confidence.

This isn't about pushing harder; it's about knowing how to troubleshoot wisely, with your long-term well-being in mind.

Why the scale sometimes "lies"

You step on the scale after a week of eating better, moving more, and staying consistent, and it barely budges. Or worse, it goes up. It feels discouraging, even confusing. But here's the truth: the scale doesn't always tell the whole story.

Your weight is influenced by far more than fat loss. Water retention, hormones, digestion, inflammation, sleep quality, and even stress levels can all affect the number you see. For example, if you've eaten more salt than usual, your body might hold on to extra water. If your muscles are sore from workouts, inflammation from recovery can temporarily add weight. These aren't setbacks, they're normal biological processes.

Building muscle (which is denser than fat) may help keep the scale steady as your body becomes leaner and stronger. That's why you might notice your clothes fitting better, your energy increasing, or your face looking slimmer, even if the number isn't moving.

This is where mindset matters. If you rely only on the scale, you might miss the real progress happening in your body and your habits. It's not lying, it's just not the whole picture.

Focus on how you feel, how you move, and how your choices are aligning with your goals. The scale is just one tool, not the ultimate judge of your success.

What to do when progress stalls

Hitting a plateau can feel like running into a wall, especially when you've been putting in the effort and doing "everything right." But here's the good news: a stall in progress is not failure. It's often a natural part of any health or wellness journey. And with a few intentional adjustments, you can move forward again, stronger and wiser.

First, pause and reflect. Are you still following your habits consistently? Over time, it's easy to slip into less mindful eating or skip a few workouts without realizing it. Revisit your routines, track your meals for a few days, or check your sleep and hydration. Minor inconsistencies can add up.

Next, mix things up. Your body is highly adaptive. If you've been doing the same exercises or eating the same foods for weeks, your metabolism may have adjusted. Try increasing the intensity or duration of your workouts, introduce strength training if you haven't already, or adjust your meal composition.

Also, zoom out. Progress isn't only about fat loss or muscle gain. Are you feeling more energized? Sleeping better? Managing stress more effectively? These changes may not be visible on the scale, but they're real wins.

Be patient and kind to yourself. Sometimes your body needs a little time to recalibrate before moving forward again. Continue to show up with consistency, and trust that results will follow.

A stall is not the end of your journey; it's a signpost asking for a slight shift. Keep going. You're still on track.

Safe weight loss for women with medical conditions

When you're managing a medical condition, whether it's PCOS, thyroid issues, diabetes, or heart concerns, weight loss can feel even more complex. But it's possible to make progress safely, without risking your health or overwhelming your system. The key is personalization, patience, and prioritizing your well-being above all else.

Before beginning any weight loss program, consult your healthcare provider. This step is not just a formality; it ensures that your approach complements any medications, therapies, or dietary restrictions you might have. Some conditions may make it harder to lose weight, but they also require extra care in how you pursue it.

Focus on nutrient-dense, anti-inflammatory foods. These not only support weight loss but also help manage inflammation, hormone balance, and energy stability. Think colorful vegetables, lean proteins, omega-3-rich fats, and low-glycemic fruits. For some women, reducing gluten or dairy intake can also make a noticeable difference; however, always consult your doctor to confirm what's appropriate for your specific condition.

Exercise should be tailored to your energy levels and physical capabilities. Gentle movements, such as walking, yoga, or light strength training, may be more sustainable than high-intensity workouts. Consistency matters more than intensity.

Lastly, monitor your progress with more than just the scale. Track how you feel in terms of your mood, digestion, sleep, and energy levels. Weight loss might come slower, but the goal is long-term health, not short-term fixes.

You deserve a plan that supports your body, not one that fights against it. Listen closely, go gently, and trust that your progress, however gradual, is still powerful.

Dealing with cravings and setbacks

Cravings and setbacks are a regular part of every woman's weight loss journey. They're not signs of failure, they're signs you're human. What matters most is how you respond when they show up.

Cravings often aren't just about food. They can be your body's way of asking for rest, comfort, hydration, or emotional release. Before you reach for that chocolate bar or salty snack, pause and ask yourself: *Am I hungry? Or am I tired, stressed, or bored?* Often, a glass of water, a short walk, or a few deep breaths can reset the moment.

That said, it's perfectly fine to enjoy the food you love. Restrictive mindsets often make cravings stronger. When you permit yourself to enjoy a treat *mindfully,* not as a reward, punishment, or escape, you reduce the guilt and regain control. Build balanced meals with fiber, protein, and healthy fats, which help curb physical cravings by stabilizing blood sugar.

As for setbacks, they happen to everyone. A missed workout, an unplanned binge, or even a few weeks off track doesn't erase your progress. It's not about being perfect; it's about staying committed even after a tough day. Look at setbacks as data, not drama. Ask yourself: *What triggered this? What could I do differently next time?*

Progress is rarely linear. Expect ups and downs, and let go of the pressure to get it "right" every single time. What builds lasting change isn't willpower; it's self-compassion, consistency, and learning from your patterns.

Cravings fade. Setbacks pass. But your commitment to yourself? That's what will carry you forward.

Navigating busy schedules and travel

Life rarely slows down when you're trying to build healthier habits. Between work, family, errands, and unexpected plans, sticking to a wellness routine can feel nearly impossible. Add travel into the mix, and it's easy to fall back into old patterns. But here's the truth: you do not need a perfect schedule or a fully stocked kitchen to make consistent progress; you need a flexible mindset and a few reliable strategies.

Start by simplifying. Instead of overhauling everything, focus on *what's realistic for you right now*. Maybe it's a 15-minute walk between meetings. Perhaps it's ordering grilled chicken and veggies instead of fast food. Perhaps it's preparing snacks for your car, office, or carry-on bag. Every small choice counts.

When your calendar is packed, **planning becomes your best friend**. Look ahead at your week. Are there two mornings when you can squeeze in movement? Can you batch-cook a simple meal to last for a few lunches? Even 10 minutes of preparation can save you hours of stress later.

Travel requires the same thoughtful approach. If you're staying in a hotel, look for one with a fitness center or bring resistance bands that fit in your suitcase. Use apps or short videos for quick in-room workouts. If eating out, scan menus online beforehand and choose a balanced option before you arrive. Keep high-protein snacks, such as almonds, protein bars, or hard-boiled eggs, on hand to avoid impulsive choices when hunger strikes.

And most importantly, **stay kind to yourself**. Travel and busy seasons are not the enemy of progress; they're a part of real life. Your goal is not to control every detail but to stay steady through the changes. If one day is off track, reset the next. If your routine shifts, adjust without judgment.

Success isn't about having a perfect schedule; it's about learning to show up for yourself *even when life is messy*. With a bit of planning, patience, and self-trust, you can keep moving forward, no matter where the day or the road takes you.

When to seek professional help

While self-guided strategies can take you far on your weight loss journey, there are times when reaching out to a professional isn't just helpful, it's necessary. Your health, both physical and emotional, deserves expert care when things feel too complex, confusing, or overwhelming to manage on your own.

Here are some signs it may be time to seek professional help:

You've hit a wall despite consistent effort. If you're doing everything "right" but not seeing results, or you're feeling constantly exhausted, moody, or unwell, it's time to consult a doctor, a registered dietitian, or a certified personal trainer. You may be dealing with hormonal imbalances, nutritional deficiencies, or an underlying medical condition that requires support beyond diet and exercise.

Your relationship with food or your body is becoming unhealthy. If you're experiencing guilt after eating, obsessively tracking calories, overexercising, or avoiding social situations because of food anxiety, a therapist, especially one who specializes in eating behavior, can help. Healing your mindset is just as important as changing your habits.

You feel lost or unmotivated. Sometimes, despite knowing what to do, you may struggle to start or maintain momentum. A coach, counselor, or support group can help you rebuild structure, confidence, and momentum. You do not have to figure it all out on your own.

Medical conditions complicate your journey. If you live with PCOS, thyroid issues, diabetes, or are recovering from childbirth or surgery, getting tailored advice from healthcare professionals ensures your efforts are safe and effective.

There is no shame in asking for help. Doing so is a sign of strength and commitment to your well-being. Think of professional support not as a last resort but as a wise investment in your long-term health.

Your journey is personal, but it doesn't have to be lonely. When the path feels too heavy to carry alone, reach out. The right guidance can make all the difference between feeling stuck and moving forward with clarity, compassion, and tangible results.

FAQ: Real women's questions answered

This section addresses the most common questions women ask during their weight loss journey, offering honest and non-judgmental answers. Whether you're just starting or fine-tuning your progress, these answers are here to support you.

Q1: Why am I gaining weight even when I'm eating healthy?

It's not always about the food. Hormones, sleep quality, stress, medication, and water retention can all impact your weight. Eating healthily is vital, but actual progress involves managing your entire lifestyle, not just calories.

Q2: I have PCOS/hypothyroidism/menopause, can I still lose weight?

Yes, but it may take a different approach. These conditions affect hormones and metabolism. Instead of extreme diets, focus on steady nutrition, blood sugar balance, strength training, and consulting a professional who understands your condition.

Q3: What if I make a mistake for a few days? Have I ruined everything?

Not. A slip-up does not erase progress. What matters most is what you do next. Be kind to yourself, reset your routine, and move forward without guilt. One choice doesn't define your whole journey.

Q4: How do I stay motivated when the scale isn't moving?

Look beyond the scale. Are you sleeping better? Feeling more energized? Less bloated? Those are real wins. Focus on non-scale victories and remember: fat loss, strength, and healing often happen before the numbers shift.

Q5: Do I have to cut carbs to lose weight?

No. Carbs are not the enemy; processed, low-nutrient carbs might be, but whole food carbs like oats, fruit, and sweet potatoes can fuel your body. Balanced meals and portion awareness are far more effective than food fear.

Q6: I'm too busy, how can I possibly stay consistent?

Start small. Prep easy meals, keep workouts short and effective, and focus on progress over perfection. Some weeks will be more complex than others. What matters is continuing to show up in ways that are realistic for your life.

Q7: What if my family or friends don't support me?

This is tough, but your journey is yours. Set boundaries when needed, communicate your goals clearly, and connect with communities (online or local) that share your mindset. Support can be found and built.

Q8: Will I have to eat like this forever?

No. The goal isn't to diet forever, it's to build a lifestyle that feels natural, enjoyable, and flexible. Once you understand what works for your body, it becomes easier to maintain without rigid rules.

CHAPTER 12

Weight Loss Recipes for Real Women

——————— ∞ ———————

Eating well does not have to mean eating bland or boring food. In this chapter, you will find simple, nourishing, and satisfying recipes created with real women — and real life — in mind. These meals are designed to support your goals without taking hours in the kitchen or requiring expensive ingredients.

From energizing breakfasts to hearty dinners and smart snacks, each recipe focuses on balanced nutrition with a practical approach. You will find meals that help manage hunger, stabilize energy, and support fat loss, without cutting out the foods you enjoy.

These recipes are flexible, family-friendly, and easy to adjust for your preferences or dietary needs. Whether you are a beginner in the kitchen or just need quick meal ideas, this chapter offers a realistic and supportive way to stay consistent with your goals — one delicious plate at a time.

Breakfasts

Greek Yogurt & Berry Parfait

A refreshing, no-fuss breakfast or snack layered with creamy yogurt and juicy berries.

Ingredients:

- 1 cup plain Greek yogurt
- ½ cup fresh strawberries, sliced
- ½ cup fresh blueberries
- 2 tablespoons granola (optional for crunch)
- 1 teaspoon honey or maple syrup (optional)

Required Tools:

- Glass or bowl
- Spoon

Instructions:

1. In a glass or small bowl, add half of the Greek yogurt.
2. Layer with half the strawberries and blueberries.
3. Add the remaining yogurt on top.
4. Finish with the remaining berries.
5. Sprinkle granola on top if using, and drizzle with honey or syrup if desired.
6. Serve immediately and enjoy.

Estimated Nutritional Information (per serving):

- Calories: ~220 kcal
- Protein: 17 g
- Carbohydrates: 25 g
- Sugars: 14 g
- Fiber: 3 g
- Fat: 6 g

Veggie Egg Muffins

A protein-packed, grab-and-go breakfast loaded with colorful vegetables — perfect for busy mornings.

Ingredients:

- 6 large eggs
- ½ cup diced bell peppers (red, green, or yellow)
- ¼ cup chopped spinach
- ¼ cup chopped onions
- ¼ cup grated low-fat cheese (optional)
- Salt and black pepper to taste
- Cooking spray or olive oil for greasing

Required Tools:

- Mixing bowl
- Whisk or fork
- Muffin tin (6 cups)
- Oven

Instructions:

1. Preheat your oven to 180°C (350°F).
2. Lightly grease a 6-cup muffin tin with cooking spray or a little olive oil.
3. In a mixing bowl, crack and whisk the eggs. Season with salt and pepper.
4. Add diced vegetables and cheese (if using) into the eggs and mix well.

5. Pour the mixture evenly into the muffin cups, filling each about ¾ full.
6. Bake for 18–20 minutes or until the muffins are firm and slightly golden on top.
7. Let cool slightly before removing. Serve warm or store in the fridge for up to 3 days.

Estimated Nutritional Information (per muffin, with cheese):

- Calories: ~90 kcal
- Protein: 7 g
- Carbohydrates: 2 g
- Sugars: 1 g
- Fiber: 0.5 g
- Fat: 6 g

Overnight Oats with Chia and Blueberries

Ingredients:

- ½ cup rolled oats
- 1 tablespoon chia seeds
- ½ cup unsweetened almond milk (or milk of choice)
- ¼ cup plain Greek yogurt
- ¼ cup fresh or frozen blueberries
- 1 teaspoon honey or maple syrup (optional)
- A pinch of cinnamon (optional)

Required Tools:

- Mason jar or airtight container

- Spoon for mixing
- Refrigerator

Instructions:

1. In a jar or container, combine oats, chia seeds, almond milk, and Greek yogurt.
2. Stir well until the mixture is smooth and even.
3. Add blueberries and a drizzle of honey or maple syrup if desired.
4. Sprinkle a pinch of cinnamon on top.
5. Seal the container and refrigerate overnight (or at least 4 hours).
6. In the morning, stir again and enjoy chilled. You can add extra berries or nuts if desired.

Estimated Nutritional Information (per serving):

- Calories: ~250 kcal
- Protein: 11 g
- Carbohydrates: 30 g
- Sugars: 7 g
- Fiber: 6 g
- Fat: 8 g

Spinach & Feta Omelette

A protein-rich, savory breakfast option that supports satiety and lean muscle maintenance—perfect for a satisfying start to your day.

Ingredients:

- 2 large eggs
- ½ cup fresh spinach, chopped
- 2 tablespoons crumbled feta cheese
- 1 tablespoon chopped onion (optional)
- Salt and black pepper to taste
- 1 teaspoon olive oil or nonstick spray

Required Tools:

- Mixing bowl
- Fork or whisk
- Non-stick skillet
- Spatula

Instructions:

1. Crack the eggs into a bowl, add a pinch of salt and pepper, and whisk until fully combined.
2. Heat olive oil in a non-stick skillet over medium heat.
3. Add chopped onion (if using) and sauté for 1–2 minutes until soft.
4. Add spinach and cook for another minute until wilted.
5. Pour in the beaten eggs and gently swirl to spread evenly across the pan.
6. Cook for 2–3 minutes or until the eggs begin to set.
7. Sprinkle feta cheese evenly over one half of the omelette.

8. Fold the omelette in half and cook for another 1–2 minutes until fully set.
9. Slide onto a plate and serve warm.

Estimated Nutritional Information (per serving):

- Calories: ~220 kcal
- Protein: 14 g
- Carbohydrates: 3 g
- Sugars: 1 g
- Fiber: 1 g
- Fat: 17 g

Apple-Cinnamon Quinoa Porridge

A warm, hearty breakfast rich in plant-based protein and fiber — ideal for cozy mornings and stable energy throughout the day.

Ingredients:

- ½ cup uncooked quinoa
- 1 cup unsweetened almond milk (or milk of choice)
- ½ cup water
- 1 small apple, peeled and diced
- ½ teaspoon ground cinnamon
- 1 teaspoon maple syrup or honey (optional)
- A pinch of salt
- Optional toppings: chopped walnuts, extra apple slices, or a sprinkle of flaxseed

Required Tools:

- Small saucepan
- Spoon or whisk
- Measuring cups and spoons
- Bowl for serving

Instructions:

1. Rinse the quinoa under cold water using a fine mesh strainer to remove its natural bitterness.
2. In a small saucepan, combine quinoa, almond milk, water, diced apple, cinnamon, and a pinch of salt.
3. Bring to a boil over medium heat, then reduce heat to low and cover.
4. Simmer for 15–20 minutes, stirring occasionally, until the quinoa is soft and the liquid is mostly absorbed.
5. If desired, stir in maple syrup or honey for a touch of sweetness.
6. Remove from heat and let sit covered for 2 minutes before serving.
7. Spoon into a bowl and top with your choice of walnuts, extra apples, or flaxseed.

Estimated Nutritional Information (per serving):

- Calories: ~260 kcal
- Protein: 7 g
- Carbohydrates: 40 g
- Sugars: 9 g
- Fiber: 5 g

- Fat: 7 g

Avocado Toast with Poached Egg

A satisfying, nutrient-dense breakfast packed with healthy fats, fiber, and protein—great for a balanced start to your day.

Ingredients:

- 1 slice whole grain or sourdough bread
- ½ ripe avocado
- 1 egg
- 1 tsp lemon juice
- Salt and pepper to taste
- Optional: red pepper flakes, cherry tomatoes, fresh herbs (like parsley or chives)

Required Tools:

- Toaster or pan for bread
- Small saucepan
- Slotted spoon
- Small bowl
- Fork
- Knife

Instructions:

1. Toast the bread until golden and crisp.
2. In a small bowl, mash the avocado with lemon juice, salt, and pepper.

3. Bring a small pot of water to a gentle simmer (not boiling).
4. Crack the egg into a small bowl. Stir the simmering water to create a gentle whirlpool, then slowly slide the egg into the center.
5. Poach the egg for 3–4 minutes, until the white is set and the yolk remains soft.
6. Remove the egg using a slotted spoon and gently pat dry with a paper towel.
7. Spread mashed avocado on the toast and top with the poached egg.
8. Sprinkle with optional toppings like red pepper flakes or fresh herbs.

Estimated Nutritional Information (per serving):

- Calories: ~290 kcal
- Protein: 10 g
- Carbohydrates: 20 g
- Sugars: 1 g
- Fiber: 6 g
- Fat: 18 g

Lunches

Lunchtime should never feel like a chore or a compromise. This chapter is all about making midday meals that keep you energized without weighing you down. These recipes are designed for real life—simple to prepare, full of flavor, and balanced to support your goals. Whether you're working from home, packing a lunchbox, or reheating something quick between errands, you'll find practical, delicious ideas here that prioritize protein, fiber, and smart carbs. Expect meals that help you stay focused and full, without relying on processed foods or diet trends. Let's make lunch a moment of care — not stress.

Grilled Chicken Salad with Mixed Greens

A fresh, protein-rich lunch that supports weight management and balanced nutrition. This salad is quick to prepare, colorful, and deeply satisfying.

Ingredients:

- 1 grilled chicken breast (approx. 120g), sliced
- 2 cups mixed salad greens (spinach, arugula, romaine)
- ½ cup cherry tomatoes, halved
- ¼ cucumber, sliced
- 1 tablespoon olive oil
- 1 teaspoon lemon juice or balsamic vinegar
- Salt and pepper to taste

Required Tools:

- Grill pan or outdoor grill
- Salad bowl
- Knife and cutting board
- Small bowl for mixing dressing

Step-by-Step Instructions:

1. **Grill the Chicken:** Lightly season the chicken breast with salt and pepper. Grill until fully cooked

(internal temp: 75°C / 165°F), about 6–7 minutes per side. Let rest for 5 minutes before slicing.
2. **Prepare Vegetables:** Wash and cut the greens, tomatoes, and cucumber.
3. **Mix Dressing:** Whisk olive oil and lemon juice or vinegar in a small bowl.
4. **Assemble:** In a large bowl, combine greens, tomatoes, cucumber, and grilled chicken. Drizzle dressing on top and toss gently.
5. **Serve:** Enjoy fresh for best texture and flavor.

Nutrient Value (Approximate per serving):

- **Calories:** 350 kcal
- **Protein:** 32g
- **Carbohydrates:** 6g
- **Fat:** 22g
- **Fiber:** 3g
- **Sugars:** 3g
- **Sodium:** 280mg

Quinoa & Chickpea Power Bowl

A fiber-rich, plant-powered lunch bowl packed with protein, whole grains, and vibrant veggies. Great for energy, digestion, and satiety — perfect for real women on a wellness journey.

Ingredients:

- ½ cup cooked quinoa
- ½ cup canned chickpeas (drained and rinsed)

- ½ avocado, sliced
- ½ cup cherry tomatoes, halved
- ¼ cup shredded red cabbage
- ½ small carrot, grated
- 1 tablespoon olive oil
- 1 teaspoon lemon juice
- Salt and pepper to taste

Required Tools:

- Small saucepan (for quinoa)
- Cutting board and knife
- Mixing bowl
- Serving bowl

Step-by-Step Instructions:

1. **Cook Quinoa:** Rinse quinoa and cook according to package instructions (usually 1 part quinoa to 2 parts water). Fluff and let cool.
2. **Prep Vegetables:** Slice avocado, tomatoes, and cabbage. Grate the carrot.
3. **Assemble the Bowl:** Add the cooked quinoa to a bowl, then top with chickpeas, veggies, and avocado.
4. **Make Dressing:** In a small bowl, mix olive oil, lemon juice, salt, and pepper.
5. **Finish:** Drizzle dressing over the bowl and serve fresh or pack for lunch.

Nutrient Value (Approximate per serving):

- **Calories:** 420 kcal
- **Protein:** 13g
- **Carbohydrates:** 35g
- **Fat:** 24g
- **Fiber:** 10g
- **Sugars:** 4g
- **Sodium:** 290mg

Tuna-Stuffed Bell Peppers

A light, protein-packed lunch that combines lean tuna with crunchy vegetables inside sweet bell peppers. Ideal for weight loss and clean eating—simple, satisfying, and easy to prepare.

Ingredients:

- 1 large bell pepper (any color), halved and seeded
- 1 (5 oz) can tuna in water, drained
- 1 tablespoon plain Greek yogurt (or light mayo)
- 1 tablespoon diced celery
- 1 tablespoon chopped red onion
- 1 teaspoon lemon juice
- Salt and pepper to taste
- Optional: chopped parsley for garnish

Required Tools:

- Mixing bowl
- Spoon

- Cutting board and knife

Step-by-Step Instructions:

1. **Prepare the Bell Pepper:** Wash and halve the pepper lengthwise. Remove seeds and membranes.
2. **Make the Filling:** In a bowl, combine tuna, Greek yogurt, celery, red onion, lemon juice, salt, and pepper. Mix well.
3. **Stuff the Peppers:** Spoon the tuna mixture into each half of the bell pepper.
4. **Serve:** Top with parsley if desired. Eat fresh or chill for a quick, portable lunch.

Nutrient Value (Approximate per serving – 2 halves):

- **Calories:** 220 kcal
- **Protein:** 26g
- **Carbohydrates:** 7g
- **Fat:** 9g
- **Fiber:** 2g
- **Sugars:** 4g
- **Sodium:** 390mg

Lentil & Vegetable Soup

A hearty, fiber-rich soup loaded with protein-packed lentils and a variety of colorful vegetables. Perfect for lunch or dinner, this comforting dish supports digestion, satiety, and weight loss goals.

Ingredients:

- 1 tablespoon olive oil
- 1 small onion, chopped
- 2 garlic cloves, minced
- 2 carrots, diced
- 2 celery stalks, diced
- 1 zucchini, diced
- 1 cup chopped spinach (fresh or frozen)
- 1 cup dry brown or green lentils, rinsed
- 1 teaspoon dried thyme
- 1 teaspoon cumin
- Salt and pepper to taste
- 5 cups vegetable broth or water
- 1 tablespoon lemon juice (optional for brightness)

Required Tools:

- Large soup pot
- Wooden spoon
- Knife and cutting board

Step-by-Step Instructions:

1. **Sauté Aromatics:** Heat olive oil in a large pot over medium heat. Add onion and garlic. Cook for 2–3 minutes until softened.
2. **Add Veggies:** Stir in carrots, celery, and zucchini. Cook for 5 minutes, stirring occasionally.
3. **Add Lentils and Broth:** Add lentils, thyme, cumin, salt, pepper, and vegetable broth. Bring to a boil.

4. **Simmer:** Reduce heat to low, cover, and simmer for 25–30 minutes or until lentils are tender.
5. **Finish:** Stir in chopped spinach and lemon juice. Simmer for another 5 minutes.
6. **Serve:** Ladle into bowls and serve hot. Keeps well in the fridge for 3–4 days.

Nutrient Value (Approximate per 1.5-cup serving):

- **Calories:** 280 kcal
- **Protein:** 16g
- **Carbohydrates:** 36g
- **Fat:** 7g
- **Fiber:** 12g
- **Sugars:** 6g
- **Sodium:** 520mg

Turkey and Avocado Wrap

This quick and satisfying wrap combines lean turkey breast with creamy avocado and fresh vegetables, offering a protein-rich, heart-healthy meal perfect for lunch or a light dinner.

Ingredients:

- 1 whole wheat tortilla (8-inch)
- 3 oz sliced roasted turkey breast (nitrate-free, preferably)
- ¼ avocado, sliced
- ¼ cup shredded lettuce
- 2 slices tomato

- 2 tablespoons hummus or Greek yogurt (optional spread)
- Salt and black pepper to taste
- A few thin slices of red onion (optional)

Required Tools:

- Cutting board
- Knife
- Spoon
- Plate for assembly

Step-by-Step Instructions:

1. **Prepare Ingredients:** Slice the avocado, tomato, and onion. Set aside.
2. **Warm the Tortilla:** Optional — lightly warm the whole wheat tortilla on a dry skillet for 15–20 seconds per side for flexibility.
3. **Assemble the Wrap:**
   - Spread hummus or Greek yogurt across the center of the tortilla.
   - Layer the turkey slices, avocado, lettuce, tomato, and onion.
   - Season lightly with salt and pepper.
4. **Wrap It Up:** Fold in the sides, then roll the tortilla tightly from the bottom.
5. **Serve:** Slice diagonally and enjoy fresh, or wrap in foil for lunch on the go.

Nutrient Value (Approximate per wrap):

- **Calories:** 330 kcal
- **Protein:** 25g
- **Carbohydrates:** 25g
- **Fat:** 15g
- **Fiber:** 6g
- **Sugars:** 3g
- **Sodium:** 620mg

Asian-Inspired Cabbage Slaw with Tofu

A crunchy, refreshing, and protein-packed dish featuring crisp cabbage, marinated tofu, and a tangy sesame-ginger dressing. Ideal for a light lunch or a satisfying side.

Ingredients:

- 1 cup shredded green cabbage
- ½ cup shredded red cabbage
- ½ medium carrot, julienned
- 1 green onion, thinly sliced
- ½ tablespoon sesame seeds
- ½ teaspoon grated fresh ginger
- 1 teaspoon low-sodium soy sauce
- 1 teaspoon rice vinegar
- 1 teaspoon sesame oil
- Juice of ½ lime
- 3 oz firm tofu, cubed and lightly pan-seared or baked
- Optional: fresh cilantro or mint for garnish

Required Tools:

- Large mixing bowl
- Cutting board and knife
- Small bowl (for dressing)
- Pan (if pan-searing tofu) or oven

Step-by-Step Instructions:

1. **Prepare Tofu:** Lightly pan-sear tofu cubes in a non-stick skillet until golden brown on all sides or bake at 375°F (190°C) for 15 minutes. Let cool.
2. **Make Dressing:** In a small bowl, mix ginger, soy sauce, sesame oil, rice vinegar, and lime juice until well combined.
3. **Combine Slaw:** In a large bowl, toss green and red cabbage, carrot, and green onion.
4. **Add Tofu and Dressing:** Add cooled tofu cubes and drizzle the dressing over the slaw. Toss gently to coat.
5. **Garnish and Serve:** Sprinkle with sesame seeds and fresh herbs, if using. Serve immediately or chill for extra flavor.

Nutrient Value (Approximate per serving):

- **Calories:** 260 kcal
- **Protein:** 13g
- **Carbohydrates:** 16g
- **Fat:** 16g
- **Fiber:** 5g
- **Sugars:** 5g

- **Sodium:** 430mg

Dinners

Dinner is your opportunity to nourish your body with wholesome, satisfying foods that support overnight recovery and prepare you for the next day. These recipes are designed to be easy to prepare, nutrient-dense, and filling—without being heavy. Whether you're winding down after a busy day or looking for something simple yet delicious, this dinner section offers balanced meals that promote weight loss while honoring real women's appetites and lifestyles. From one-pan dishes to comforting bowls, each recipe provides a blend of lean protein, fiber, and healthy fats to help you feel full and supported without guilt or restriction.

Baked Salmon with Roasted Asparagus

A simple, flavorful dinner packed with protein, omega-3s, and fiber. Perfect for a nourishing, low-carb evening meal that feels both light and satisfying.

Ingredients:

- 1 salmon fillet (about 150–170g)
- 1 tsp olive oil
- 1 clove garlic, minced
- Juice of ½ lemon
- Salt and pepper to taste
- 1 cup asparagus spears, trimmed
- ½ tsp dried herbs (like dill, thyme, or Italian seasoning)

Required Tools:

- Baking sheet
- Parchment paper or foil
- Small bowl
- Oven

Instructions:

1. **Preheat the oven** to 200°C (400°F). Line a baking sheet with parchment or foil.
2. **Place the salmon** on one side of the sheet. Rub with olive oil, garlic, lemon juice, salt, pepper, and herbs.
3. **Arrange asparagus** on the other side of the tray. Drizzle with a touch of olive oil and season lightly.
4. **Bake for 12–15 minutes**, or until salmon flakes easily and asparagus is tender.
5. Serve immediately with an optional wedge of lemon.

Usage and Portioning:
One serving for an adult. This meal is great for dinner and can be paired with a small sweet potato or quinoa if more energy is needed.

Nutrient Value (Approximate per serving):

- Calories: 320
- Protein: 30g
- Fat: 20g
- Carbohydrates: 5g
- Fiber: 2g
- Omega-3s: High

Zucchini Noodles with Turkey Meatballs

A delicious low-carb twist on traditional spaghetti and meatballs. Zucchini noodles (zoodles) keep it light, while lean turkey meatballs provide satisfying protein for a balanced, weight-loss-friendly dinner.

Ingredients:
For the meatballs:

- 250g lean ground turkey
- 1 egg
- 2 tbsp finely chopped onion
- 1 garlic clove, minced
- 2 tbsp oats or almond flour (optional binder)
- Salt, pepper, and Italian seasoning to taste

For the zucchini noodles:

- 2 medium zucchinis, spiralized
- 1 tsp olive oil
- ½ cup low-sugar tomato sauce
- Fresh basil for garnish (optional)

Required Tools:

- Frying pan or skillet
- Spiralizer or julienne peeler
- Mixing bowl
- Baking tray (optional for oven method)

Instructions:

1. In a bowl, mix all meatball ingredients. Form into small balls.

2. Cook meatballs in a lightly oiled pan over medium heat for 10–12 minutes, turning occasionally until cooked through.
    (Alternatively, bake at 200°C/400°F for 15–18 minutes.)
3. In another pan, sauté zucchini noodles in 1 tsp olive oil for 2–3 minutes until just tender.
4. Warm the tomato sauce and combine with meatballs.
5. Serve meatballs over zucchini noodles. Garnish with fresh basil if desired.

Usage and Portioning:
Serves one adult. Ideal for dinner or post-workout meals. For meal prep, multiply ingredients accordingly.

Nutrient Value (Approximate per serving):

- Calories: 330
- Protein: 28g
- Fat: 18g
- Carbohydrates: 10g
- Fiber: 3g
- Sugar: 4g
- Net carbs: ~7g

Grilled Shrimp Tacos with Mango Salsa

These vibrant shrimp tacos offer a fresh, zesty flavor with a sweet and spicy mango salsa. Packed with lean protein and healthy fats, they're a refreshing and satisfying dinner that supports your weight loss goals without sacrificing flavor.

Ingredients:
For the shrimp:

- 150g shrimp, peeled and deveined
- 1 tsp olive oil
- Juice of ½ lime
- ½ tsp chili powder
- ½ tsp garlic powder
- Salt and pepper to taste

For the mango salsa:

- ½ ripe mango, diced
- 2 tbsp red onion, finely chopped
- 1 tbsp fresh cilantro, chopped
- ½ small red chili (optional), finely chopped
- Juice of ½ lime

To assemble:

- 2 small corn tortillas (or lettuce leaves for low-carb)
- ¼ avocado, sliced (optional)
- Shredded cabbage or lettuce (optional base)

Required Tools:

- Grill pan or outdoor grill
- Mixing bowls
- Knife and chopping board

Instructions:

1. Toss shrimp with olive oil, lime juice, chili powder, garlic powder, salt, and pepper. Let marinate for 10 minutes.

2. Grill shrimp over medium-high heat for 2–3 minutes per side, until opaque and cooked through.
3. In a bowl, combine mango, red onion, cilantro, red chili, and lime juice to make the salsa.
4. Warm the tortillas slightly in a pan.
5. Assemble the tacos: add shrimp, spoon over mango salsa, top with avocado and shredded greens if desired.

Nutrient Value (Approximate per serving – 2 tacos):

- Calories: 350
- Protein: 28g
- Fat: 14g
- Carbohydrates: 24g
- Fiber: 5g
- Sugar: 9g
- Net carbs: ~19g

Stir-Fried Chicken and Broccoli

Ingredients:

- 150g boneless, skinless chicken breast, thinly sliced
- 1 cup broccoli florets
- 1 tbsp low-sodium soy sauce
- 1 tsp sesame oil (or olive oil)
- 1 tsp fresh ginger, grated
- 1 garlic clove, minced
- 1 tsp cornstarch (optional, for thickening)
- 2 tbsp water

Required Tools:

- Non-stick skillet or wok

- Knife and chopping board
- Mixing bowl

Instructions:

1. In a bowl, mix soy sauce, water, cornstarch (if using), ginger, and garlic to make the sauce.
2. Heat sesame oil in a pan over medium-high heat.
3. Add chicken slices and cook until browned and cooked through (about 5–6 minutes).
4. Remove chicken and set aside.
5. Add broccoli to the same pan with a splash of water. Stir-fry for 3–4 minutes until tender-crisp.
6. Return the chicken to the pan and pour in the sauce. Cook for 1–2 more minutes, stirring until everything is coated.

Usage and Portioning:
Serves one adult as a full dinner. Serve with a small portion of brown rice or cauliflower rice if desired.

Nutrient Value (Approximate per serving):

- Calories: 290
- Protein: 32g
- Fat: 10g
- Carbohydrates: 14g
- Fiber: 3g
- Sugar: 3g
- Net carbs: ~11g

Cauliflower Rice Veggie Stir-Fry

A light, low-carb alternative to traditional fried rice, this colorful veggie stir-fry with cauliflower rice is packed with fiber, flavor, and nutrients. It's ideal for dinner or meal prep when you want something satisfying without feeling heavy.

Ingredients:

- 1½ cups cauliflower rice (fresh or frozen)
- ½ cup diced bell pepper (any color)
- ½ cup chopped zucchini
- ¼ cup shredded carrots
- ¼ cup chopped red onion
- 1 garlic clove, minced
- 1 tbsp low-sodium soy sauce (or coconut aminos)
- 1 tsp sesame oil or olive oil
- Optional: 1 scrambled egg or ¼ cup edamame for added protein

Required Tools:

- Non-stick skillet or wok
- Grater or food processor (if using fresh cauliflower)
- Spatula

Instructions:

1. Heat sesame oil in a skillet over medium heat.
2. Add garlic and red onion; sauté for 1–2 minutes.
3. Add bell pepper, zucchini, and carrots. Stir-fry for 3–4 minutes.
4. Stir in cauliflower rice and soy sauce. Cook for 4–5 minutes until tender but not mushy.
5. If using, mix in scrambled egg or edamame in the last 2 minutes.
6. Taste and adjust seasoning if needed.

Usage and Portioning:
Serves one adult as a light dinner or hearty lunch. Can be

doubled for batch cooking or served with grilled tofu, shrimp, or chicken for added protein.

Nutrient Value (Approximate per serving without added protein):

- Calories: 160
- Protein: 4g
- Fat: 7g
- Carbohydrates: 17g
- Fiber: 5g
- Sugar: 6g
- Net Carbs: ~12g

One-Pan Lemon Herb Chicken & Veggies

This simple one-pan dinner is a complete, balanced meal featuring juicy lemon-herb chicken breast, roasted vegetables, and minimal cleanup. It's perfect for busy weeknights or meal prep with lean protein, fiber-rich veggies, and vibrant flavor.

Ingredients:

- 1 skinless, boneless chicken breast (approx. 5–6 oz)
- ½ cup chopped zucchini
- ½ cup chopped bell peppers (any color)
- ½ cup broccoli florets
- 1 tbsp olive oil
- Juice of ½ lemon
- 1 tsp dried oregano
- ½ tsp garlic powder
- Salt and pepper to taste

Required Tools:

- Baking sheet
- Parchment paper or non-stick spray
- Mixing bowl
- Oven

Instructions:

1. Preheat oven to 400°F (200°C). Line a baking sheet with parchment paper.
2. In a bowl, toss chicken breast and vegetables with olive oil, lemon juice, oregano, garlic powder, salt, and pepper.
3. Spread evenly on the baking sheet, keeping chicken in the center and veggies around it.
4. Bake for 20–25 minutes or until the chicken is cooked through (internal temp 165°F) and veggies are tender.
5. Optional: Broil for the last 2–3 minutes for a lightly crisp finish.

Usage and Portioning:
Serves one adult as a full dinner. Easily scaled up for family meals or weekly meal prep. Store leftovers in an airtight container for up to 3 days.

Nutrient Value (Approximate per serving):

- Calories: 320
- Protein: 35g
- Fat: 14g
- Carbohydrates: 14g
- Fiber: 4g
- Sugar: 5g
- Net Carbs: ~10g

Snacks & Light Bites

Snacking does not have to derail your health goals — in fact, when done right, it can support steady energy, reduce cravings, and keep your metabolism active between meals. In this section, you will find smart, satisfying snack ideas that are quick to prepare, portion-friendly, and aligned with a balanced weight loss lifestyle. Whether you need a post-workout boost, a mid-morning nibble, or a healthy evening treat, these recipes are designed to nourish without the guilt. Each snack offers a mix of protein, fiber, and healthy fats to keep you full and fueled throughout your day.

Hummus & Raw Veggie Sticks

A crunchy, creamy, and satisfying snack packed with fiber, healthy fats, and plant-based protein. Perfect for curbing afternoon cravings or enjoying as a light bite before dinner.

Ingredients:

- ½ cup hummus (store-bought or homemade)
- 1 small carrot, sliced into sticks
- 1 celery stalk, cut into sticks
- ½ cucumber, sliced
- ½ bell pepper, sliced

Required Tools:

- Cutting board
- Knife
- Small serving bowl or container

Preparation Instructions:

1. Wash and slice all the vegetables into easy-to-dip sticks.
2. Portion hummus into a small bowl or lunch container.
3. Arrange the veggie sticks around the hummus or pack separately if on the go.

Usage and Portioning:
This recipe serves one adult. It makes a great midday snack or a colorful appetizer when entertaining.

Nutrient Value (approximate):

- Calories: 210
- Protein: 6g
- Fat: 11g
- Carbohydrates: 22g
- Fiber: 7g

Cottage Cheese with Pineapple

A sweet and savory combo that's refreshing, protein-rich, and perfect for a mid-morning or post-workout snack. This balanced snack helps support muscle recovery while keeping you satisfied.

Ingredients:

- ½ cup low-fat cottage cheese
- ½ cup pineapple chunks (fresh or canned in juice, drained)

Required Tools:

- Spoon
- Small bowl or container

Preparation Instructions:

1. Add cottage cheese to a bowl.
2. Top with pineapple chunks.
3. Mix gently if preferred, or keep layered for texture contrast.
4. Serve chilled.

Usage and Portioning:
Serves one adult. This recipe works well as a light snack, breakfast side, or dessert replacement.

Nutrient Value (approximate):

- Calories: 150
- Protein: 13g
- Fat: 2g
- Carbohydrates: 18g
- Fiber: 1g

Spicy Roasted Chickpeas

A crunchy, satisfying, high-protein snack that curbs cravings without the guilt. These roasted chickpeas are seasoned to perfection and ideal for on-the-go snacking or movie night munching.

Ingredients:

- 1 can (15 oz) chickpeas, drained and rinsed
- 1 tablespoon olive oil

- ½ teaspoon smoked paprika
- ¼ teaspoon cayenne pepper (adjust to taste)
- ½ teaspoon garlic powder
- ¼ teaspoon sea salt

Required Tools:

- Baking sheet
- Parchment paper (optional)
- Mixing bowl
- Spoon

Preparation Instructions:

1. Preheat oven to 400°F (200°C).
2. Pat chickpeas dry with a paper towel for extra crispiness.
3. In a bowl, toss chickpeas with olive oil and spices until evenly coated.
4. Spread on a baking sheet in a single layer.
5. Roast for 25–30 minutes, shaking halfway through, until crispy and golden brown.
6. Let cool before serving (they continue to crisp as they cool).

Usage and Portioning:
Yields approximately 2 servings. Store leftovers in an airtight container for up to 3 days.

Nutrient Value (per serving, approx.):

- Calories: 180
- Protein: 7g
- Fat: 6g
- Carbohydrates: 24g
- Fiber: 6g

Protein-Packed Energy Balls

These no-bake energy balls are the perfect blend of protein, healthy fats, and fiber — ideal for a post-workout snack or a mid-day energy boost. They're easy to make, portable, and naturally sweetened.

Ingredients:

- 1 cup rolled oats
- ½ cup natural peanut butter (or almond butter)
- ¼ cup honey or maple syrup
- ¼ cup mini dark chocolate chips
- 2 tablespoons chia seeds
- 2 tablespoons flaxseed meal
- 1 scoop protein powder (vanilla or chocolate, optional)
- 1 teaspoon vanilla extract
- Pinch of salt

Required Tools:

- Mixing bowl
- Spoon or spatula
- Measuring cups
- Baking sheet or plate for chilling

Preparation Instructions:

1. In a large bowl, mix all ingredients until well combined.
2. Use your hands or a spoon to form the mixture into 1-inch balls.
3. Place on a lined plate or tray and refrigerate for 20–30 minutes to firm up.

4. Store in an airtight container in the fridge for up to 1 week.

Usage and Portioning:
Makes approximately 12 energy balls. One serving = 2 balls.

Nutrient Value (per serving of 2 balls, approx.):

- Calories: 220
- Protein: 8g
- Fat: 11g
- Carbohydrates: 22g
- Fiber: 4g

Apple Slices with Almond Butter

A simple yet satisfying snack, apple slices with almond butter provide a balanced combination of natural sugars, healthy fats, and fiber. It's a great go-to option for curbing sweet cravings while staying on track with your weight loss goals.

Ingredients:

- 1 medium apple (any variety)
- 2 tablespoons almond butter (unsweetened, smooth or crunchy)

Required Tools:

- Sharp knife
- Cutting board
- Small bowl or plate

Preparation Instructions:

1. Wash and core the apple, then slice it into thin wedges.
2. Spread almond butter on each slice or serve it on the side as a dip.
3. Optional: Sprinkle a pinch of cinnamon or chia seeds on top for extra flavor and nutrition.

Usage and Portioning:
Serves one adult as a light snack. Perfect for mid-morning or afternoon energy boost.

Nutrient Value (approximate):

- Calories: 200
- Protein: 4g
- Fat: 12g
- Carbohydrates: 22g
- Fiber: 5g

Edamame with Sea Salt

Ingredients:

- 1 cup edamame in pods (fresh or frozen)
- 1/4 teaspoon sea salt (adjust to taste)

Preparation Instructions:

1. Bring water to a boil in a saucepan or steamer.
2. Add edamame and cook for 4–5 minutes until tender but still firm.
3. Drain and transfer to a bowl.
4. Sprinkle sea salt while hot and toss to coat evenly.

5. Serve warm or cold — simply squeeze the beans from the pod with your teeth.

Nutrient Value (approximate per 1 cup cooked edamame):

- Calories: 190
- Protein: 18g
- Fat: 8g
- Carbohydrates: 14g
- Fiber: 8g

CHAPTER 13

4-Week Meal Plan for Weight Loss

--------------------- ·✕· ---------------------

This plan is not about perfection or restriction. It's about simplicity, nourishment, and creating lasting habits. You'll find a balanced mix of breakfasts, lunches, dinners, and snacks that are easy to prepare, affordable, and full of flavor. Each week is structured to reduce decision fatigue and keep you on track without the stress. Whether you're a beginner or restarting your journey, this plan will help you stay consistent while honoring your hunger, energy, and lifestyle. Let's make healthy eating doable one meal at a time.

How to use the meal plan for your goals

This 4-week meal plan is a flexible tool designed to support your weight loss journey in a sustainable, enjoyable way. It's not about strict dieting or punishing rules; it's about learning to fuel your body with intention, ease, and joy.

To make it work for you:

1. Start With Your Why

Before you begin, take a moment to revisit your personal goals. Are you here to lose weight? Build healthier habits?

Feel more energized in your day-to-day life? Knowing your "why" helps you stay motivated and grounded when life gets busy or cravings sneak in.

2. Stick to the Structure, Not Perfection

Each day includes:

- Breakfast
- Lunch
- Dinner
- One to Two Snacks

Feel free to adjust based on your appetite and schedule. If you skip a snack or switch lunch with dinner, it's completely okay. The goal is consistency, not rigidity.

3. Mix & Match When Needed

If you find a meal you love, repeat it. If something doesn't appeal to you, swap it out with another option from the same category (e.g., replace one lunch with another lunch). The recipes are intentionally interchangeable within the plan.

4. Portion Mindfully

The meals are crafted for one adult serving, with options to double or triple for family or meal prep. Portion size matters. Listen to your hunger and fullness cues, and resist the urge to over-restrict or overeat. Intuitive eating is part of long-term success.

5. Prep in Advance

Use your weekends or a free evening to prep ingredients, wash and chop veggies, cook grains or proteins, or pre-pack snacks. Even 30 minutes of prep can make your week smoother and less stressful.

6. Hydrate Daily

Aim for at least 6–8 glasses of water per day, especially if you're increasing fiber or activity levels. Hydration helps digestion, reduces bloating, and keeps your energy steady.

7. Track How You Feel, Not Just What You Eat

Consider journaling your mood, sleep, energy levels, and digestion. Progress isn't just about the scale; it's about how your body feels, functions, and responds.

This plan is meant to support, not control, you. If you miss a day or eat outside the plan, return to your next meal with intention. Progress is built one bite, one choice, and one day at a time.

Customizing for dietary preferences/allergies

Your body, your rules. This meal plan is not one-size-fits-all, and it shouldn't be. Whether you are vegetarian, dairy-free, gluten-sensitive, or have dietary restrictions, everything in this plan can be adjusted to meet your needs without sacrificing balance or taste.

1. Vegetarian or Vegan?

- **Protein swaps**: Replace chicken, turkey, or fish with tofu, tempeh, seitan, or legumes like lentils and chickpeas.
- **Egg-free breakfasts**: Try chia pudding, plant-based smoothies, or oatmeal with nut butter.
- **Dairy-free alternatives**: Use unsweetened almond, oat, or coconut milk, and plant-based yogurts or cheeses.

2. Gluten-Free Adjustments

Swap whole-grain bread, wraps, or pasta for certified gluten-free versions like rice noodles, quinoa pasta, or lettuce wraps.

- Replace soy sauce with tamari or coconut aminos.
- Check labels on condiments and dressings; gluten can hide in surprising places.

3. Dairy-Free Modifications

- Use coconut or almond yogurt instead of Greek yogurt.
- Try nutritional yeast in place of cheese for a savory, cheesy flavor.
- Swap regular milk for plant-based milk in porridges, smoothies, or baking.

4. Nut Allergies

- Replace almond butter with sunflower seed or pumpkin seed butter.

- Avoid nuts in salads or snacks, use seeds or crunchy roasted chickpeas for texture.
- Always read labels on protein bars or energy bites.

5. Low-Carb/Keto Tweaks

- Skip grains like quinoa, oats, or brown rice and substitute with cauliflower rice, zoodles, or leafy greens.
- Add more healthy fats like olive oil, avocado, and seeds.
- Stick to non-starchy vegetables and moderate protein portions.

6. Picky Eater Tips

- Don't like broccoli? Try spinach, zucchini, or bell peppers.
- Texture-sensitive? Blend veggies into sauces or soups.
- Keep seasoning bold or straightforward, depending on your taste preferences.

Always listen to your body. If something doesn't sit right digestively, energetically, or emotionally, change it. The best eating plan is one that makes you feel nourished, safe, and satisfied. This guide is a blueprint, not a rulebook. You're in charge.

Meal Plan Table

Day	Breakfast	Lunch	Dinner	Snack(s)
1	Greek Yogurt & Berry Parfait	Grilled Chicken Salad	Baked Salmon with Roasted Asparagus	Apple Slices with Almond Butter
2	Overnight Oats with Chia & Blueberries	Quinoa & Chickpea Power Bowl	Zucchini Noodles with Turkey Meatballs	Hummus & Raw Veggie Sticks
3	Veggie Egg Muffins	Tuna-Stuffed Bell Peppers	Stir-Fried Chicken and Broccoli	Cottage Cheese with Pineapple
4	Spinach & Feta Omelette	Lentil & Vegetable Soup	Grilled Shrimp Tacos with Mango Salsa	Protein-Packed Energy Balls
5	Apple-Cinnamon Quinoa Porridge	Turkey and Avocado Wrap	Cauliflower Rice Veggie Stir-Fry	Edamame with Sea Salt
6	Avocado Toast with Poached Egg	Asian-Inspired Cabbage Slaw with Tofu	One-Pan Lemon Herb Chicken & Veggies	Spicy Roasted Chickpeas
7	Greek	Grilled	Baked	Apple

Day	Breakfast	Lunch	Dinner	Snack(s)
	Yogurt & Berry Parfait	Chicken Salad	Salmon with Roasted Asparagus	Slices with Almond Butter
8	Overnight Oats with Chia & Blueberries	Quinoa & Chickpea Power Bowl	Zucchini Noodles with Turkey Meatballs	Hummus & Raw Veggie Sticks
9	Veggie Egg Muffins	Tuna-Stuffed Bell Peppers	Stir-Fried Chicken and Broccoli	Cottage Cheese with Pineapple
10	Spinach & Feta Omelette	Lentil & Vegetable Soup	Grilled Shrimp Tacos with Mango Salsa	Protein-Packed Energy Balls
11	Apple-Cinnamon Quinoa Porridge	Turkey and Avocado Wrap	Cauliflower Rice Veggie Stir-Fry	Edamame with Sea Salt
12	Avocado Toast with Poached Egg	Asian-Inspired Cabbage Slaw with Tofu	One-Pan Lemon Herb Chicken & Veggies	Spicy Roasted Chickpeas
13	Greek Yogurt & Berry Parfait	Grilled Chicken Salad	Baked Salmon with Roasted Asparagus	Apple Slices with Almond Butter

Day	Breakfast	Lunch	Dinner	Snack(s)
14	Overnight Oats with Chia & Blueberries	Quinoa & Chickpea Power Bowl	Zucchini Noodles with Turkey Meatballs	Hummus & Raw Veggie Sticks
15	Veggie Egg Muffins	Tuna-Stuffed Bell Peppers	Stir-Fried Chicken and Broccoli	Cottage Cheese with Pineapple

Weekly shopping list and prep tips

Produce

- Apples (6–8)
- Bananas (optional for smoothies/snacks)
- Berries (blueberries, strawberries, raspberries – 4 cups total)
- Spinach (fresh or frozen – 4 cups)
- Mixed greens or lettuce (2 large bags)
- Avocados (6)
- Bell peppers (4–6 mixed colors)
- Cucumber (2)
- Cherry tomatoes (2 cups)
- Broccoli (2 heads or bags)
- Zucchini (4)
- Carrots (6)
- Asparagus (2 bunches)
- Red cabbage (½ head or bagged slaw mix)
- Mango (2, or 1 cup frozen chunks)
- Lemons (2)

- Garlic (1 bulb)
- Onions (yellow and red – 4–5 total)
- Fresh herbs (parsley, cilantro, or dill – optional)

Proteins

- Eggs (1–2 dozen)
- Greek yogurt, plain unsweetened (32 oz)
- Cottage cheese, low-fat (16 oz)
- Chicken breasts, boneless skinless (4–6 pieces)
- Ground turkey (1 lb)
- Canned tuna in water (2 cans)
- Shrimp, peeled and deveined (1–1.5 lb)
- Salmon fillets (2–4)
- Tofu (firm – 1 block)
- Lentils (dried or canned – 2 cups cooked)
- Chickpeas (canned or dried – 2 cups cooked)
- Edamame, shelled (frozen – 1 bag)

Grains & Legumes

- Rolled oats (2 cups)
- Chia seeds (½ cup)
- Quinoa (1–2 cups)
- Brown rice or cauliflower rice (1 bag or 2 cups cooked)
- Whole wheat wraps (4–6)
- Low-sugar granola (optional – 1 cup)
- Whole grain bread (1 loaf)

Pantry Items

- Olive oil or avocado oil
- Apple cider vinegar
- Balsamic vinegar
- Soy sauce or coconut aminos
- Mustard or Dijon
- Nut butter (almond or peanut – unsweetened)
- Low-sodium broth (vegetable or chicken)
- Canned tomatoes (1 can)
- Salt, pepper, and dried herbs/spices (e.g., cumin, paprika, garlic powder)

Snacks & Extras

- Hummus (store-bought or homemade)
- Protein powder (optional for energy balls)
- Dark chocolate chips (optional for snacks)
- Nuts/seeds (almonds, walnuts, sunflower seeds – 1–2 cups total)

Weekly Prep Tips

1. Batch Cook Proteins:

- Grill or bake chicken breasts for salads and wraps.
- Prepare turkey meatballs and freeze in portions.
- Hard-boil 6–8 eggs for quick breakfasts or snacks.

2. Make Breakfasts Ahead:

- Prepare overnight oats for 3–4 days.

- Bake a batch of veggie egg muffins and refrigerate or freeze.
- Pre-portion Greek yogurt + berries into jars.

3. Chop Veggies in Advance:

- Dice onions, bell peppers, cucumbers, and carrots.
- Store in airtight containers for quick use during the week.

4. Cook Grains in Batches:

- Cook quinoa, brown rice, or cauliflower rice in bulk.
- Store in containers to use in bowls or stir-fries.

5. Make Dressings & Hummus:

- Mix a simple vinaigrette or tahini dressing and store in a mason jar.
- Prep homemade hummus for snacks and wraps.

Flexibility for busy weeks

Life doesn't always stick to a schedule, and neither should your wellness plan. Whether you're juggling work meetings, parenting duties, or unexpected errands, your weight loss journey can and should flex with you. A busy week doesn't mean failure. It simply means finding more innovative ways to keep going.

Start by letting go of the all-or-nothing mindset. If you cannot follow your exact meal plan or fit in a full workout, that's okay. Progress happens in the small choices too, like choosing water over soda, taking the stairs instead of the elevator, or eating a home-prepped wrap instead of fast food. These moments count.

Tips for Staying on Track During Hectic Times:

- **Meal Prep Light**: If a full prep session is too much, chop some veggies, boil a few eggs, and stock easy proteins like Greek yogurt, hummus, and canned tuna.
- **Stock the Freezer**: Keep healthy, homemade meals in the freezer, such as soup, turkey meatballs, or veggie stir-fry. Just heat and serve.
- **Snack Smart**: Keep portioned snacks like almonds, roasted chickpeas, or protein balls in your bag or car so you're not caught off guard when hunger strikes.
- **Choose Efficient Workouts**: A 10-minute brisk walk, stretching session, or bodyweight circuit at home still moves your body and supports your mindset.
- **Stay Connected**: When things get hectic, check in with your support system, a friend, a coach, or even a journal. A few minutes to reset can help you stay focused.

Permit yourself to adapt. One imperfect week will not undo your results. What matters is staying in motion, even when it's not perfect. Flexibility is not a weakness; it's a superpower in real-life wellness.

How to Adjust Portion Sizes

Portion control is not about restriction; it's about balance. Understanding how much your body truly needs can make the difference between constant frustration and sustainable progress. Learning to adjust portion sizes based on your hunger, activity level, and specific weight loss goals is an empowering skill, not a rulebook.

Start with Visual Cues

You don't always need a scale or measuring cups to get it right. Use these everyday objects as visual references:

Food Type	Portion Size	Visual Cue
Protein (meat, tofu)	3–4 oz cooked	Size of your palm
Vegetables	1 cup cooked / 2 cups raw	Size of your two fists
Carbs (rice, pasta)	½ to 1 cup cooked	Size of a cupped hand
Healthy Fats	1 tbsp (nut butter, oil)	Tip of your thumb
Cheese	1 oz	Size of a pair of dice
Fruit	1 medium piece or ½ cup sliced	Size of your fist

Adjust Based on Your Goals

- **If you're losing too slowly**: Slightly reduce starchy carbs and added fats first, not protein or veggies.
- **If you're too hungry**: Increase fiber-rich foods like beans or veggies to feel fuller longer.
- **For active days**: Add extra carbs (like brown rice or sweet potato) post-workout to help your body recover.

Listen to Your Body

Mindful eating supports portion control. Pause halfway through your meal to check in: Are you still truly hungry, or just eating out of habit? It's okay to stop when satisfied and save the rest. Leftovers are your friend.

Keep It Flexible

Not every meal needs to be "perfect." The goal is to eat portions that nourish you and keep your energy steady, not leave you drained or overly full. Portion control works best when it's consistent, not rigid.

With practice, portioning becomes intuitive. It's less about counting and more about awareness, an essential step toward long-term health and freedom with food.

CHAPTER 14

25 Essential Weight Loss Exercises

—————— ∞ ——————

Weight loss is not just about what you eat; how you move matters too. This chapter brings together 25 essential exercises that support fat burning, muscle toning, and overall body confidence. These moves are handpicked to fit real women's lives, no fancy gym memberships or extreme routines required.

Whether you're a beginner starting from scratch or looking to level up your current workouts, you'll find a mix of cardio, strength, and flexibility exercises that can be done at home or on the go. Each one includes guidance on form, duration, and modifications so you can feel strong, safe, and supported every step of the way.

Bodyweight Strength Exercises

Bodyweight exercises are a convenient, effective way to build strength, tone muscles, and boost metabolism without needing any equipment. These movements rely on your own body as resistance, making them accessible anywhere at home, in a park, or while traveling. Beyond burning calories, bodyweight exercises improve posture, balance, and core stability, helping you move more efficiently in everyday life. In this section, you'll learn foundational moves that target major muscle groups and can be adapted for any fitness level, providing a solid base for lasting strength and confidence.

Bodyweight Squat

A foundational lower-body exercise that strengthens the quadriceps, hamstrings, glutes, and core. Perfect for building functional strength and supporting weight loss.

Required Tools:

- None (bodyweight only)
- Optional: yoga mat for comfort

Step-by-Step Instructions:

- Stand with your feet shoulder-width apart, toes slightly pointing outward.
- Engage your core and keep your chest lifted.
- Slowly bend your knees and push your hips back as if sitting into a chair.
- Lower down until your thighs are parallel to the floor (or as far as comfortable).
- Keep your weight on your heels and avoid letting your knees extend past your toes.
- Press through your heels to return to the starting position.
- Repeat for 10–15 reps for beginners, or adjust based on your fitness level.

Safety Measures:

- Maintain a neutral spine; do not round your lower back.
- Keep knees aligned with toes to prevent joint strain.
- Avoid bouncing or jerking movements; perform squats in a slow, controlled manner.
- Stop immediately if you feel sharp pain in your knees, hips, or lower back.
- Warm up your lower body before starting your session.

Push-Up

A classic upper-body exercise that strengthens the chest, shoulders, triceps, and core while improving overall stability.

Required Tools:

- None (bodyweight only)
- Optional: yoga mat or soft surface for comfort

Step-by-Step Instructions:

1. Start in a high plank position with your hands slightly wider than shoulder-width apart and your feet hip-width apart.
2. Engage your core, keeping your back flat and hips in line with your shoulders.
3. Slowly bend your elbows and lower your chest toward the floor while keeping your body straight.

4. Lower until your chest is just above the ground (or as far as comfortable).
5. Push through your palms to straighten your arms and return to the starting position.
6. Repeat for 8–15 reps depending on your fitness level.

Safety Measures:

- Keep your core tight to prevent sagging hips or arching your back.
- Avoid flaring your elbows too wide; aim for a 45-degree angle from your body.
- Perform the movement slowly and controlled to avoid shoulder strain.
- If standard push-ups are too challenging, modify by lowering your knees to the floor.
- Stop immediately if you experience sharp pain in your shoulders, wrists, or back.

Glute Bridge

A lower-body exercise that targets the glutes, hamstrings, and core while improving hip stability and posture. Ideal for strengthening the posterior chain and enhancing functional movement.

Required Tools:

- None (bodyweight only)
- Optional: yoga mat for comfort

Step-by-Step Instructions:

1. Lie on your back with knees bent and feet flat on the floor, hip-width apart.
2. Place your arms by your sides with palms facing down.
3. Engage your core and squeeze your glutes as you lift your hips toward the ceiling.
4. Continue lifting until your body forms a straight line from shoulders to knees.
5. Hold the position for 1–2 seconds, then slowly lower your hips back to the starting position.
6. Repeat for 12–15 reps for beginners, adjusting reps as needed.

Safety Measures:

- Keep your core engaged to prevent arching your lower back.
- Avoid lifting your hips too high, which can strain your lower back.
- Press through your heels to activate the glutes rather than overusing your lower back.
- Perform the movement in a slow, controlled manner to maximize effectiveness.
- Stop immediately if you feel discomfort or sharp pain in your back or hips.

Lunge (Forward and Reverse)

A versatile lower-body exercise that strengthens the quadriceps, hamstrings, glutes, and calves while improving balance and stability. Both forward and reverse lunges engage the core for better overall control.

Required Tools:

- None (bodyweight only)
- Optional: yoga mat for comfort

Step-by-Step Instructions:

Forward Lunge:

- Stand upright with feet hip-width apart and hands on your hips or at your sides.
- Step forward with your right foot, lowering your hips until both knees are bent at approximately 90 degrees.
- Ensure your front knee is directly above your ankle and your back knee hovers just above the floor.
- Press through your front heel to return to the starting position.
- Repeat with the left leg. Alternate for 10–12 reps per leg.

Reverse Lunge:

- Stand upright with feet hip-width apart.
- Step backward with your right foot, lowering your hips until both knees are bent at approximately 90 degrees.
- Keep your torso upright and core engaged.
- Press through your front heel to return to the starting position.

- Repeat with the left leg. Alternate for 10–12 reps per leg.

Safety Measures:

- Maintain a straight torso throughout the movement; do not lean forward.
- Keep knees aligned with toes to avoid joint strain.
- Perform movements slowly and in a controlled manner; avoid jerking motions.
- Do not let your front knee extend past your toes.
- Stop immediately if you experience sharp pain in your knees, hips, or lower back.

Tricep Dip (Chair or Bench)

This is an effective upper-body exercise that targets the triceps, shoulders, and chest. Ideal for strengthening the arms and improving functional pushing strength.

Required Tools:

- Stable chair, bench, or low table
- Optional: yoga mat for cushioning

Step-by-Step Instructions:

1. Sit on the edge of the chair or bench with your hands gripping the edge, fingers facing forward, and feet flat on the floor.
2. Slide your hips forward off the chair so that your hands and feet support your weight.

3. Keep your elbows close to your body and bend them to lower your hips toward the floor until your elbows reach about a 90-degree angle.
4. Press through your palms to straighten your arms and lift your body back to the starting position.
5. Repeat for 10–15 reps, maintaining controlled movement throughout.

Safety Measures:

- Ensure the chair or bench is stable and won't slide during the exercise.
- Keep your shoulders down and away from your ears to prevent strain.
- Avoid locking your elbows at the top of the movement.
- Move slowly and control your range of motion; do not bounce.
- Stop immediately if you feel pain in your shoulders, wrists, or elbows.

Wall Sit

A static lower-body exercise that targets the quadriceps, glutes, and core. Wall sits build endurance and strength, making them ideal for supporting weight loss and overall lower-body stability.

Required Tools:

- Wall or flat vertical surface
- Optional: yoga mat for back comfort

Step-by-Step Instructions:

1. Stand with your back flat against a wall, feet shoulder-width apart, and about 2 feet away from the wall.
2. Slide your back down the wall while bending your knees, lowering your body until your thighs are parallel to the floor (like sitting in an invisible chair).
3. Keep your knees directly above your ankles and avoid letting them extend past your toes.
4. Engage your core and glutes, keeping your back pressed against the wall.
5. Hold the position for 20–60 seconds, depending on your fitness level.
6. Slowly slide back up the wall to stand and rest before repeating for 2–3 sets.

Safety Measures:

- Maintain a neutral spine and avoid arching your lower back.
- Keep weight evenly distributed on your heels, not toes.
- Do not allow knees to collapse inward; keep them aligned with your toes.
- Breathe steadily; avoid holding your breath during the hold.
- Stop immediately if you experience sharp pain in your knees, lower back, or hips.

Plank

A core-strengthening exercise that targets the abdominals, lower back, shoulders, and glutes. Planks improve posture, stability, and overall functional strength—essential for weight loss and daily movement.

Required Tools:

- Yoga mat or soft surface for comfort
- Optional: timer

Step-by-Step Instructions:

Forearm Plank:

1. Lie face down on the mat and place your forearms on the ground, elbows directly under your shoulders.
2. Engage your core and lift your body so it forms a straight line from head to heels.
3. Keep your hips level, avoid sagging or lifting them too high.
4. Hold the position for 20–60 seconds, breathing steadily throughout.
5. Lower gently to the mat and rest before repeating for 2–3 sets.

Full (High) Plank:

- Start in a push-up position with your hands directly under your shoulders and arms fully extended.

- Keep your body in a straight line from head to heels, engaging your core and glutes.
- Avoid letting your lower back sag or your hips rise.
- Hold for 20–60 seconds, then rest. Repeat for 2–3 sets.

Safety Measures:

- Maintain a neutral spine; do not let your lower back sag.
- Keep shoulders stacked over elbows or wrists, depending on plank type.
- Engage the core and glutes throughout to protect the lower back.
- Avoid holding the plank if you experience pain in your shoulders, wrists, or lower back.
- Start with shorter holds and gradually increase duration as your strength improves.

Side Plank

A core-focused exercise that targets the obliques, shoulders, and glutes. Side planks improve stability, balance, and functional strength while enhancing overall core definition.

Required Tools:

- Yoga mat or soft surface for comfort
- Optional: timer

Step-by-Step Instructions:

1. Lie on your side with your legs extended, stacking your feet one on top of the other.
2. Place your bottom elbow directly under your shoulder, forearm flat on the mat.
3. Engage your core and lift your hips off the ground, forming a straight line from head to feet.
4. Keep your top arm either resting on your hip or extended straight toward the ceiling for balance.
5. Hold the position for 15–45 seconds, depending on your fitness level.
6. Slowly lower your hips back to the mat and switch sides.
7. Repeat for 2–3 sets per side.

Safety Measures:

- Keep your body in a straight line; avoid letting your hips drop or rotate forward/backward.
- Engage the core and glutes to maintain stability.
- Align your elbow directly under your shoulder to protect the joint.
- Avoid holding the plank if you feel sharp pain in the shoulder, elbow, or lower back.
- Modify by bending the bottom knee for extra support if needed.

Mountain Climber

A dynamic, full-body exercise that combines cardio and core strengthening. Mountain climbers boost heart rate, burn calories, and engage the abs, shoulders, and legs simultaneously.

Required Tools:

- Yoga mat or soft surface for comfort
- Optional: timer

Step-by-Step Instructions:

1. Start in a high plank position with your hands directly under your shoulders and body forming a straight line from head to heels.
2. Engage your core and bring your right knee toward your chest.
3. Quickly switch legs, bringing your left knee toward your chest while extending your right leg back.
4. Continue alternating legs in a controlled, rhythmic motion, keeping your hips level.
5. Perform for 20–40 seconds per set, depending on your fitness level, or complete 10–20 reps per leg.
6. Rest briefly and repeat for 2–3 sets.

Safety Measures:

- Keep your core tight to avoid sagging hips or arching your back.
- Maintain shoulders stacked over wrists to prevent joint strain.
- Move in a controlled manner; avoid bouncing or jerking motions.
- Stop immediately if you experience pain in your wrists, shoulders, or lower back.

- Modify by slowing down the movement or stepping one leg at a time if needed.

Bird Dog

A core and stability exercise that targets the abdominals, lower back, glutes, and shoulders. Bird dogs improve balance, spinal alignment, and functional strength.

Required Tools:

- Yoga mat or soft surface for comfort

Step-by-Step Instructions:

1. Begin on all fours with your hands directly under your shoulders and knees under your hips.
2. Engage your core to keep your spine neutral.
3. Slowly extend your right arm straight forward while simultaneously extending your left leg straight back.
4. Keep your hips and shoulders square to the floor.
5. Hold for 2–3 seconds, then slowly return to the starting position.
6. Repeat with your left arm and right leg.
7. Perform 8–12 reps per side for 2–3 sets.

Safety Measures:

- Keep movements slow and controlled to avoid straining the lower back.
- Engage the core throughout to maintain spinal alignment.

- Avoid arching or sagging your back during the movement.
- Stop immediately if you feel discomfort in the shoulders, hips, or lower back.
- Modify by extending only the arm or leg if full extension is challenging.

Step-Up (Stairs or Bench)

A functional lower-body exercise that targets the quadriceps, glutes, hamstrings, and calves. Step-ups improve balance, stability, and cardiovascular endurance while supporting weight loss and functional strength.

Required Tools:

- Sturdy bench, step, or set of stairs
- Optional: dumbbells for added resistance
- Optional: yoga mat for cushioning

Step-by-Step Instructions:

1. Stand facing the bench or step with feet hip-width apart.
2. Step onto the bench with your right foot, pressing through your heel to lift your body upward.
3. Bring your left foot to meet the right, standing fully upright on the bench.
4. Step back down with your left foot first, followed by your right foot, to return to the starting position.
5. Repeat for 10–12 reps per leg, alternating leading leg if desired.

6. Perform 2–3 sets, adjusting reps or adding weight as your strength improves.

Safety Measures:

- Ensure the step or bench is stable and secure before performing the exercise.
- Keep your chest lifted and core engaged throughout the movement.
- Avoid leaning excessively forward or backward to protect your knees and lower back.
- Step fully with the entire foot on the platform to prevent slipping.
- Stop immediately if you experience pain in your knees, hips, or lower back.

Cardio & Fat-Burning Moves

Cardio exercises are a cornerstone of any weight loss journey. These movements elevate your heart rate, increase calorie burn, and improve cardiovascular health while boosting energy and endurance. In this chapter, you'll find a variety of fat-burning exercises that can be performed at home, outdoors, or in the gym — no special equipment required. From high-intensity bursts to steady-paced routines, each exercise is designed to maximize calorie expenditure, strengthen your muscles, and support long-term weight management. These moves are adaptable for all fitness levels, giving you the tools to move confidently and efficiently toward your goals.

Jumping Jacks

A classic full-body cardio exercise that raises your heart rate, burns calories, and improves cardiovascular endurance. Jumping jacks also engage the legs, core, and shoulders, making them an excellent fat-burning move.

Required Tools:

- None (bodyweight only)
- Optional: yoga mat or soft surface for comfort

Step-by-Step Instructions:

1. Stand upright with your feet together and arms at your sides.
2. Jump both feet out to the sides while simultaneously raising your arms overhead.
3. Quickly return to the starting position with feet together and arms at your sides.
4. Continue at a steady, controlled pace.
5. Perform for 30–60 seconds per set, or complete 20–30 repetitions.
6. Repeat for 2–3 sets depending on your fitness level.

Safety Measures:

- Land softly on the balls of your feet to reduce impact on your knees.
- Keep your core engaged to protect your lower back.
- Move in a controlled rhythm; avoid locking your knees.

- Stop immediately if you feel sharp pain in the knees, hips, or shoulders.
- Modify by stepping one foot out at a time instead of jumping if needed.

High Knees

A dynamic cardio move that elevates heart rate, burns calories, and strengthens the legs and core. High knees improve endurance, coordination, and lower-body power while supporting fat loss.

Required Tools:

- None (bodyweight only)
- Optional: yoga mat or cushioned surface for comfort

Step-by-Step Instructions:

1. Stand tall with feet hip-width apart and arms at your sides.
2. Engage your core and lift your right knee toward your chest while simultaneously driving your left arm forward.
3. Quickly switch, lifting your left knee and moving your right arm forward, maintaining a running-in-place motion.
4. Continue alternating knees at a fast, controlled pace.
5. Perform for 20–40 seconds per set, or complete 30–50 repetitions per leg.
6. Repeat for 2–3 sets depending on your fitness level.

Safety Measures:

- Land softly on the balls of your feet to reduce stress on knees and ankles.
- Keep your core engaged and back straight to prevent lower-back strain.
- Avoid locking your knees; maintain a slight bend during impact.
- Move in a controlled rhythm; do not overstride or lean forward.
- Stop immediately if you experience sharp pain in your knees, hips, or lower back.

Burpees

A full-body, high-intensity exercise that combines strength and cardio. Burpees boost heart rate, burn calories, and engage multiple muscle groups, including arms, chest, core, glutes, and legs.

Required Tools:

- None (bodyweight only)
- Optional: yoga mat for cushioning

Step-by-Step Instructions:

1. Stand upright with feet shoulder-width apart and arms at your sides.
2. Lower into a squat, placing your hands on the floor in front of you.
3. Jump your feet back into a high plank position, keeping your body straight.

4. Perform a push-up (optional for beginners; can skip).
5. Jump your feet forward toward your hands, returning to the squat position.
6. Explosively jump up, reaching your arms overhead.
7. Land softly and immediately go into the next repetition. Perform 8–12 reps for beginners or adjust based on fitness level.

Safety Measures:

- Maintain a neutral spine during the plank and push-up portions.
- Land softly to reduce impact on knees and ankles.
- Move in a controlled manner; avoid rushing and compromising form.
- Modify by eliminating the push-up or jumping step if necessary.
- Stop immediately if you feel pain in your wrists, shoulders, knees, or lower back.

March in Place

A low-impact cardio exercise that increases heart rate, improves circulation, and warms up the body. Marching in place is suitable for beginners and can be used as a warm-up or active recovery move.

Required Tools:

- None (bodyweight only)

- Optional: comfortable shoes and a yoga mat for cushioning

Step-by-Step Instructions:

1. Stand tall with feet hip-width apart and arms relaxed at your sides.
2. Lift your right knee toward your chest while swinging your left arm forward.
3. Lower your right leg and simultaneously lift your left knee, swinging your right arm forward.
4. Continue alternating knees in a marching motion at a controlled pace.
5. Perform for 1–3 minutes per set, or adjust duration based on your fitness level.
6. Increase Intensity by lifting knees higher or moving faster as your endurance improves.

Safety Measures:

- Keep your core engaged and back straight to maintain proper posture.
- Land gently on your feet to reduce impact on knees and ankles.
- Avoid leaning forward or backward; maintain an upright position.
- Stop immediately if you experience discomfort in your hips, knees, or lower back.
- Modify by taking smaller steps if balance or knee issues are present.

Skater Jumps

A dynamic, lateral cardio exercise that strengthens the legs, glutes, and core while improving balance, agility, and cardiovascular fitness. Skater jumps mimic a skating motion for a fun, high-intensity movement.

Required Tools:

- None (bodyweight only)
- Optional: yoga mat for cushioning

Step-by-Step Instructions:

1. Stand with feet hip-width apart, knees slightly bent, and core engaged.
2. Push off your right foot and jump laterally to the left, landing on your left foot.
3. Bring your right foot behind your left leg without touching the ground, like a skating motion.
4. Swing your arms naturally to maintain balance.
5. Immediately push off the left foot and jump laterally to the right, repeating the motion.
6. Perform 10–15 jumps per side for beginners, adjusting reps or sets as needed.

Safety Measures:

- Land softly on the balls of your feet to reduce impact on knees and ankles.
- Keep a slight bend in your knees when landing to absorb shock.
- Engage your core to maintain balance and prevent twisting the lower back.

- Move in a controlled manner to avoid falls or ankle strain.
- Stop immediately if you feel pain in your knees, hips, or lower back.

Jump Rope

A high-intensity cardio exercise that improves cardiovascular fitness, coordination, and agility while burning calories efficiently. Jump rope can be adapted to all fitness levels for fat-burning and endurance building.

Required Tools:

- Jump rope (adjustable length recommended)
- Flat, non-slip surface
- Optional: yoga mat or cushioned flooring for joint protection

Step-by-Step Instructions:

1. Hold the jump rope handles firmly in each hand, with the rope behind your heels.
2. Stand with feet together, elbows close to your body, and core engaged.
3. Swing the rope over your head and jump as it passes under your feet, landing softly on the balls of your feet.
4. Maintain a consistent rhythm, keeping your jumps low to reduce joint impact.
5. Perform continuously for 30–60 seconds per set or complete 50–100 jumps depending on your fitness level.

6. Rest for 30–60 seconds between sets; repeat for 2–4 sets.

Safety Measures:

- Keep your core engaged and back straight to avoid leaning forward.
- Land softly with knees slightly bent to protect joints.
- Use proper rope length to prevent tripping.
- Wear supportive shoes to cushion your feet and ankles.
- Stop immediately if you feel sharp pain in your feet, knees, or lower back.

Butt Kicks

A dynamic cardio exercise that targets the hamstrings, glutes, and calves while boosting heart rate. Butt kicks are great for warming up, improving flexibility, and burning calories.

Required Tools:

- None (bodyweight only)
- Optional: yoga mat or cushioned surface for comfort

Step-by-Step Instructions:

1. Stand tall with feet hip-width apart and arms relaxed at your sides.
2. Engage your core and begin jogging in place.

3. As you lift each leg, bring your heel up toward your glutes in a kicking motion.
4. Pump your arms naturally as you move to maintain rhythm.
5. Continue alternating legs at a steady, controlled pace.
6. Perform for 30–60 seconds per set or complete 20–40 kicks per leg, repeating for 2–3 sets.

Safety Measures:

- Land softly on the balls of your feet to reduce impact on knees and ankles.
- Maintain an upright posture and keep your core engaged to protect the lower back.
- Move in a controlled rhythm to avoid overstraining hamstrings.
- Stop immediately if you feel pain in your knees, calves, or lower back.
- Modify by reducing speed or range of motion if necessary.

Standing Side Crunch

A core-focused exercise that targets the obliques and strengthens the lateral abdominal muscles. Standing side crunches also engage the hips and improve balance and posture.

Required Tools:

- None (bodyweight only)
- Optional: yoga mat for comfort or stability

Step-by-Step Instructions:

1. Stand upright with feet shoulder-width apart and hands behind your head, elbows out to the sides.
2. Engage your core and lift your right knee toward your right elbow while bending your torso slightly to the right.
3. Slowly return to the starting position.
4. Repeat on the left side, lifting your left knee toward your left elbow.
5. Alternate sides for 10–15 repetitions per side.
6. Perform 2–3 sets depending on your fitness level.

Safety Measures:

- Keep your movements slow and controlled to prevent strain on your lower back.
- Avoid pulling on your neck with your hands; let the core do the work.
- Maintain an upright posture and avoid leaning forward.
- Stop immediately if you feel sharp pain in your lower back, hips, or neck.
- Modify by reducing the range of motion if full side crunches are too challenging.

Core & Flexibility

A strong core and flexible body are essential for overall fitness, weight loss, and injury prevention. Core strength supports proper posture, stabilizes the spine, and improves performance in both daily activities and workouts. Flexibility, meanwhile, enhances range of motion, reduces muscle tension, and allows your body to move more efficiently. In this chapter, you'll find exercises that target the abdominal muscles, obliques, lower back, and hips while incorporating stretches and movements to improve flexibility. These exercises are designed for all fitness levels and can be adapted to your pace, helping you feel stronger, more agile, and balanced in your body.

Bicycle Crunch

A dynamic abdominal exercise that targets the rectus abdominis, obliques, and hip flexors. Bicycle crunches improve core strength, stability, and coordination while helping tone the midsection.

Required Tools:

- Yoga mat or soft surface for comfort

Step-by-Step Instructions:

1. Lie flat on your back with your hands lightly behind your head, elbows wide.
2. Lift your knees to a 90-degree angle and bring your shins parallel to the floor.
3. Engage your core and lift your shoulders slightly off the ground.
4. Rotate your torso to bring your right elbow toward your left knee while extending your right leg straight.
5. Switch sides, bringing your left elbow toward your right knee while extending your left leg straight.

6. Continue alternating sides in a slow, controlled cycling motion for 10–20 reps per side.
7. Perform 2–3 sets depending on your fitness level.

Safety Measures:

- Keep movements slow and controlled to avoid neck or lower-back strain.
- Avoid pulling on your neck with your hands; focus on engaging your abdominal muscles.
- Maintain a neutral lower back pressed gently against the mat.
- Stop immediately if you feel sharp pain in your neck, back, or hips.
- Modify by reducing the range of motion or keeping the shoulders on the mat if needed.

Russian Twist

A core-strengthening exercise that targets the obliques, abdominals, and lower back. Russian twists improve rotational strength, stability, and balance while engaging the entire midsection.

Required Tools:

- Yoga mat or soft surface for comfort
- Optional: small weight, medicine ball, or water bottle for added resistance

Step-by-Step Instructions:

1. Sit on the floor with your knees bent and feet flat on the ground.

2. Lean back slightly while keeping your back straight and core engaged.
3. Clasp your hands together or hold a weight in front of your chest.
4. Lift your feet slightly off the ground for more challenge (optional).
5. Rotate your torso to the right, bringing your hands or weight beside your hip.
6. Return to the center, then rotate to the left side.
7. Continue alternating sides for 12–20 reps per side. Perform 2–3 sets depending on your fitness level.

Safety Measures:

- Keep your core tight to protect your lower back.
- Move in a controlled manner; avoid jerky rotations.
- Do not round your back; maintain a straight spine throughout.
- Stop immediately if you feel pain in your lower back, shoulders, or hips.
- Modify by keeping your feet on the floor for added stability if needed.

Leg Raise

A core-focused exercise that targets the lower abdominals and hip flexors. Leg raises help build core strength, improve stability, and enhance overall abdominal definition.

Required Tools:

- Yoga mat or soft surface for comfort

Step-by-Step Instructions:

1. Lie flat on your back with your legs extended and arms by your sides or under your glutes for support.
2. Engage your core and lift both legs toward the ceiling, keeping them straight.
3. Slowly lower your legs toward the floor without letting your lower back arch off the mat.
4. Stop just before your feet touch the ground and lift them back up to the starting position.
5. Perform 10–15 repetitions per set. Repeat for 2–3 sets depending on your fitness level.

Safety Measures:

- Keep your lower back pressed gently against the mat to avoid strain.
- Move in a slow, controlled manner; avoid jerking the legs.
- Engage your core throughout the movement for stability.
- Stop immediately if you feel pain in your lower back, hips, or shoulders.
- Modify by bending your knees slightly if full-leg raises are too challenging.

Standing Oblique Crunch

A core-strengthening exercise that targets the oblique muscles, helping tone the sides of the abdomen while improving balance and stability.

Required Tools:

- None (bodyweight only)
- Optional: yoga mat for cushioning or stability

Step-by-Step Instructions:

1. Stand upright with feet hip-width apart and hands behind your head, elbows pointing outward.
2. Engage your core and lift your right knee toward your right elbow, bringing your torso slightly toward the side of the knee.
3. Lower your leg and return to the starting position.
4. Repeat on the left side, lifting your left knee toward your left elbow.
5. Continue alternating sides for 10–15 repetitions per side.
6. Perform 2–3 sets depending on your fitness level.

Safety Measures:

- Avoid pulling on your neck; let your abs do the work.
- Maintain an upright posture and keep movements slow and controlled.
- Stop immediately if you experience pain in the lower back, hips, or neck.
- Modify by reducing the range of motion if full side crunches are too challenging.

Seated Torso Twist

A flexibility and core exercise that targets the obliques, spine, and shoulders. Seated torso twists improve rotational mobility, posture, and overall core strength.

Required Tools:

- A chair or a stable surface to sit on
- Optional: yoga mat for floor version

Step-by-Step Instructions:

1. Sit upright with feet flat on the floor and knees bent at 90 degrees.
2. Cross your arms over your chest or place your hands behind your head.
3. Engage your core and slowly rotate your torso to the right as far as comfortable.
4. Return to the center, then rotate to the left.
5. Continue alternating sides for 10–15 repetitions per side.
6. Perform 2–3 sets depending on your fitness level.

Safety Measures:

- Keep your spine straight; avoid rounding your back.
- Move slowly and controlled to prevent dizziness or strain.
- Engage your core throughout to protect your lower back.
- Stop immediately if you experience pain in the spine, hips, or shoulders.

- Modify by reducing the range of motion if needed for comfort or flexibility limitations.

Cat-Cow Stretch

A gentle flexibility exercise that mobilizes the spine, stretches the back and abdominal muscles, and improves posture. Ideal for warming up, cooling down, or relieving tension in the spine.

Required Tools:

- Yoga mat or soft surface for comfort

Step-by-Step Instructions:

1. Start on all fours with your wrists directly under your shoulders and knees under your hips.
2. **Cat Pose:** Exhale and round your spine toward the ceiling, tucking your chin toward your chest and drawing your belly button in.
3. **Cow Pose:** Inhale and arch your back, lifting your chest and tailbone toward the ceiling, letting your belly drop toward the floor.
4. Flow between Cat and Cow poses slowly and gently, coordinating your breath with movement.
5. Repeat the sequence for 8–12 rounds, moving at a comfortable pace.

Safety Measures:

- Move gently; avoid forcing your spine into extreme positions.

- Keep wrists directly under shoulders to prevent strain.
- Engage your core lightly to protect the lower back.
- Stop immediately if you experience sharp pain in your back, wrists, or neck.
- Modify by placing a folded towel under your knees for extra cushioning if needed.

Warm-up and cool-down basics

Warming up and cooling down are essential components of any effective exercise routine, yet they are often overlooked. A proper warm-up prepares your body for movement by increasing blood flow to muscles, raising your core temperature, and improving joint mobility. It reduces the risk of injury and helps you perform exercises with better form and efficiency.

A cool-down, on the other hand, helps your body gradually return to a resting state. It supports recovery, prevents dizziness, and reduces post-workout muscle stiffness. Effective cool-downs often include light cardio, stretching, and breathing exercises to relax both muscles and mind

In this section, you'll learn simple, practical warm-up and cool-down strategies that can be adapted to any workout style or fitness level. By consistently including these steps, you'll enhance performance, reduce injury risk, and feel more balanced in your body before, during, and after exercise.

How to combine exercises for any fitness level

Creating an effective workout routine doesn't require a gym full of equipment or complex planning. The key is combining exercises in a way that challenges your body, supports fat loss, and builds strength while matching your current fitness level.

1. Assess Your Fitness Level

- **Beginner:** Focus on bodyweight exercises and low-impact cardio. Keep sets shorter and movements controlled.
- **Intermediate:** Include moderate-intensity cardio, strength moves with light weights, and core stability exercises.
- **Advanced:** Incorporate high-intensity intervals, compound lifts, and dynamic movements for full-body engagement.

2. Structure Your Workouts

- **Warm-Up:** 5-10 minutes of light cardio and mobility exercises to prepare joints and muscles.
- **Cardio & Fat-Burning Moves:** Select 2-4 exercises (jumping jacks, high knees, mountain climbers) performed for 30-60 seconds each, with short rest periods.
- **Strength Training:** Choose 4-6 exercises targeting major muscle groups (bodyweight squats, push-ups, lunges, glute bridges). Perform 10-15 reps per exercise or 20-40 seconds for isometric holds like wall sits or planks.

- **Core & Flexibility:** Include 2–4 exercises (bicycle crunches, side planks, stretches) to improve posture, mobility, and core strength.
- **Cool-Down:** Finish with 5–10 minutes of stretching and deep breathing to aid recovery.

3. Adjust Intensity

- Modify movements to match your strength and endurance. For example, perform knee push-ups instead of full push-ups, or step instead of jumping for low-impact cardio.
- Increase Intensity gradually by adding sets, reps, or resistance as your fitness improves.

4. Listen to Your Body

- Pay attention to fatigue, form, and discomfort. Rest or modify exercises when needed.
- Progress is measured by consistency, endurance, and strength gains, not by pushing through pain.

By combining exercises thoughtfully, you create a balanced, adaptable routine that works for beginners and advanced exercisers alike, helping you safely achieve your weight loss and fitness goals.

Adapting for home or gym

You don't need a fancy gym to get a great workout, but having access to equipment can add variety and Intensity. This section helps you adapt your exercise routine to your environment, whether you're working out at home or in a gym.

Home Workouts

Bodyweight Exercises: Squats, lunges, push-ups, planks, glute bridges, and step-ups require no equipment and can be performed in small spaces.

Simple Tools: Resistance bands, dumbbells, or kettlebells add extra challenge and variety without taking up much space.

Flexibility: Cardio can include jumping jacks, high knees, mountain climbers, or jump rope. Core and stretching exercises need only a mat.

Gym Workouts

- **Machines & Free Weights:** Use resistance machines, dumbbells, and barbells to target specific muscle groups more effectively.
- **Cardio Equipment:** Treadmills, ellipticals, stationary bikes, and rowing machines offer structured cardiovascular workouts.
- **Variety & Intensity:** Access to heavier weights and more equipment allows for progressive overload, higher resistance, and interval training.

Tips for Both Settings

- **Focus on Form:** Proper technique is more important than equipment. Maintain control and alignment in every exercise.
- **Modify as Needed:** Replace gym-specific moves with home alternatives and vice versa. For

example, a wall sit can replace a leg press machine; resistance band rows can replace cable rows.

- **Mix & Match:** Combine bodyweight, cardio, and weight-based exercises to create a balanced routine.
- **Consistency Over Equipment:** Your results depend more on regular practice than having access to the "perfect" gym setup.

By adapting exercises to your environment, you can maintain progress, stay motivated, and make your workouts both practical and effective, whether at home or in a fully equipped gym.

CHAPTER 15

Navigating Social & Family Life While Losing Weight

———— ∞ ————

Losing weight doesn't happen in isolation; it happens in the context of your everyday life, surrounded by family, friends, and social events. This chapter focuses on strategies for staying consistent with your goals while still enjoying meals, celebrations, and gatherings. You'll learn how to handle peer pressure, manage portion control in social settings, and create supportive environments at home. By approaching social and family life thoughtfully, you can maintain your progress without feeling deprived or disconnected, and build habits that are both sustainable and enjoyable in the long term.

Eating healthy at social gatherings

Social events, whether birthdays, weddings, or casual dinners, can feel challenging when you're trying to maintain healthy habits. The key is planning, awareness, and making choices that align with your goals without feeling restricted.

Practical Tips:

Survey Before You Serve: Take a quick look at what's available before filling your plate. Prioritize vegetables, lean proteins, and whole grains as your first choices.

Portion Wisely: Use a smaller plate if possible, and take smaller portions of high-calorie foods. Enjoy them mindfully rather than skipping entirely.

Eat Beforehand: Having a light, healthy snack before a party can reduce temptation and prevent overeating.

Choose Wisely: Opt for foods that nourish and satisfy rather than simply filling your stomach. Balance indulgences with nutrient-dense options.

Stay Hydrated: Drink water or sparkling water between beverages to help control hunger and prevent overeating.

Mindful Indulgence: It's okay to enjoy a treat, focus on quality, savor every bite, and avoid guilt.

By approaching social gatherings with a plan and mindful awareness, you can enjoy yourself, connect with others, and stay on track with your weight loss goals. Social life and healthy habits can coexist without compromising each other.

Managing family meal times

Family meals are important for connection and tradition, but they can also be challenging when trying to maintain healthy eating habits. The goal is to create a balance that allows you to honor your weight loss journey while still participating in shared meals.

Practical Strategies:

- **Plan Ahead:** Prepare balanced meals in advance that include lean proteins, vegetables, and whole grains. Having healthy options ready helps you avoid last-minute temptations.
- **Include Everyone:** Create recipes that the whole family can enjoy, adjusting only portion sizes or specific ingredients to accommodate your personal goals.
- **Control Portions:** Serve yourself first or use a smaller plate to help manage portion sizes without affecting others.
- **Mindful Eating:** Eat slowly, savor flavors, and listen to your body's fullness cues. Encourage conversation and connection to focus less on just the food.
- **Healthy Swaps:** Substitute ingredients in family recipes to make them more nutritious, like using whole-grain pasta, baking instead of frying, or reducing added sugars.
- **Stay Consistent:** While it's okay to enjoy favorite dishes occasionally, maintain your regular eating habits most of the time to reinforce healthy routines.

By planning, communicating, and making thoughtful choices, you can navigate family meals with confidence, enjoy quality time together, and stay committed to your weight loss goals without stress or conflict.

Staying on track during holidays

Holidays are often filled with indulgent meals, desserts, and celebrations, making it challenging to stick to your weight loss goals. However, with mindful planning and a flexible approach, you can enjoy the festivities without derailing your progress.

Practical Tips:

- **Plan:** Check menus or plan your meals to identify healthier options and avoid impulsive choices.
- **Portion Control:** Allow yourself to enjoy favorite holiday treats in moderation. Small portions help you savor the flavor without overindulging.
- **Prioritize Protein and Vegetables:** Fill most of your plate with lean proteins and colorful vegetables before adding higher-calorie items.
- **Stay Active:** Incorporate movement into your holiday routine by walking after meals, participating in family activities, or scheduling quick workouts.
- **Mindful Eating:** Eat slowly, pay attention to hunger and fullness cues, and focus on enjoying the company as much as the food.
- **Hydrate Wisely:** Drink water throughout the day, which helps with satiety and reduces unnecessary snacking.
- **Flexible Mindset:** Accept that one meal or event won't ruin progress. Return to your routine afterward without guilt.

- By combining planning, moderation, and mindfulness, you can enjoy holiday celebrations while maintaining consistency and control over your weight loss journey.

Dealing with peer pressure and food pushers

Social situations can create pressure to eat foods that don't align with your weight loss goals. Friends, family, or colleagues may unintentionally encourage overindulgence, making it challenging to stay on track. Learning strategies to handle these situations can help you maintain confidence and consistency.

Practical Strategies:

- **Be Polite but Firm:** Practice simple responses, such as "I'm good for now" or "I'm focusing on my healthy choices today." A kind, confident tone usually works best.
- **Bring Your Dish:** If attending gatherings, contribute a healthy option that you enjoy. This ensures there's something on the table that supports your goals.
- **Focus on Socializing:** Shift attention from food to conversation, games, or activities. Engaging fully with people reduces mindless eating.
- **Set Boundaries:** Decide ahead of time what you will and won't eat, and stick to your plan. It's okay to say no without feeling guilty.

- **Plan Ahead:** Eat a balanced snack before social events to reduce temptation and prevent overeating out of hunger.
- **Mindful Indulgence:** If you choose to indulge, do so consciously and in moderation. Enjoy the taste fully, then return to your usual healthy routine.
- **Positive Self-Talk:** Remind yourself why your goals are important and reinforce your ability to make choices that support your health.

By using these techniques, you can navigate peer pressure with ease, enjoy social situations, and stay committed to your weight loss journey without conflict or guilt.

Making your goals visible and fun

Turning your weight loss goals into something tangible and enjoyable can boost motivation and accountability. When you see your progress and reminders of your goals every day, it's easier to stay consistent and celebrate small wins along the way.

Practical Strategies:

- **Visual Reminders:** Place sticky notes, vision boards, or printed photos of your goals in areas you see frequently, such as the fridge, mirror, or workspace.
- **Progress Tracking:** Use a journal, planner, or mobile app to record workouts, meals, or body measurements. Tracking creates a sense of achievement.

- **Gamify Your Goals:** Turn milestones into challenges or rewards, like earning a new workout outfit after reaching a weekly target.
- **Celebrate Small Wins:** Recognize every step forward, whether it's drinking more water, completing a workout, or resisting unnecessary snacks.
- **Involve Friends or Family:** Share your goals with supportive people who can cheer you on, join you for workouts, or provide accountability.
- **Fun Challenges:** Create mini-challenges, such as "10,000 steps per day" or "3 new healthy recipes this week," to keep routines engaging.

Making your goals visible and enjoyable, you transform your weight loss journey from a chore into an engaging, motivating experience. This approach reinforces consistency, encourages positive habits, and helps you stay committed for the long term.

Quick recipes for parties and events

Maintaining healthy eating habits doesn't mean missing out on social events or celebrations. With a few innovative strategies and quick recipes, you can enjoy parties while staying aligned with your weight loss goals. The key is preparation, creativity, and balance.

Practical Strategies:

- **Mini Veggie Platters:** Cut colorful vegetables, such as bell peppers, carrots, cucumbers, and cherry tomatoes, into bite-sized pieces. Pair with a light dip, such as hummus or a Greek yogurt-based dressing.

- **Protein-Packed Finger Foods:** Offer options such as turkey or chicken skewers, hard-boiled eggs, or mini stuffed peppers. These satisfy hunger and stabilize blood sugar.
- **Fruit-Based Snacks:** Serve fresh fruit skewers, melon balls, or berries for a naturally sweet treat with minimal added sugar.
- **Whole-Grain Options:** Prepare small portions of whole-grain crackers with low-fat cheese or avocado spread for balanced snacking.
- **Simple Wraps and Rolls:** Use lettuce leaves or whole-grain tortillas to create mini wraps with lean protein and veggies — perfect for easy grabbing and eating.
- **Portion-Friendly Desserts:** Serve small servings of Greek yogurt parfaits or chia puddings to offer a healthy, visually appealing dessert option.

By choosing quick, nutritious, and portion-controlled recipes, you can enjoy social gatherings guilt-free. These options help you stay consistent with your goals while providing variety, flavor, and ease of preparation, ensuring that parties and events remain enjoyable without compromising your progress.

Role modeling for children and loved ones

Your actions speak louder than words. By demonstrating healthy habits, you can inspire those around you, especially children, to make positive lifestyle choices. Role modeling is a powerful way to reinforce the behaviors you want your family and loved ones to adopt, creating a supportive environment for everyone.

Practical Strategies:

- **Lead by Example:** Show consistency in your meals, exercise routines, and hydration habits. Children and family members are more likely to follow when they see you practicing what you preach.
- **Involve Them in Activities:** Encourage family walks, bike rides, or home workouts to get them involved. Making fitness a shared experience can turn healthy habits into enjoyable routines.
- **Cook Together:** Involve children in meal planning and preparation. Teaching them to choose and prepare balanced meals fosters lifelong skills.
- **Positive Language:** Focus on health and energy rather than appearance or weight. Emphasize feeling strong, energized, and capable.
- **Celebrate Successes:** Acknowledge achievements, no matter how small, and share the joy of progress with your loved ones.
- **Maintain Balance:** Model moderation by enjoying treats occasionally while prioritizing nutritious choices, showing that a healthy lifestyle is flexible and sustainable.

By consciously modeling healthy behaviors, you establish a positive family culture centered on food, fitness, and wellness. Your example can motivate children and loved ones to embrace habits that support long-term health and happiness.

CHAPTER 16

Weight Loss and Women's Health at Every Age

—— ∞ ——

Weight loss and overall health are not one-size-fits-all, especially for women. Hormonal changes, metabolism shifts, and lifestyle factors all influence how your body responds to diet and exercise at different stages of life. This chapter examines the distinct considerations for weight management during young adulthood, midlife, and beyond, offering personalized guidance on nutrition, exercise, and self-care tailored to each phase. By understanding your body's changing needs, you can make informed choices, maintain your energy, and achieve sustainable results, regardless of your age.

Unique Challenges in Your 20s, 30s, 40s, 50s, and Beyond

Women face different physical and lifestyle challenges at each stage of life, and understanding these changes can help tailor your weight loss and health strategies for lasting results.

20s: Establishing Habits

- Often, it's a time of busy schedules, social events, and career beginnings.

- Metabolism is typically faster, but inconsistent routines and late-night eating can impact progress.
- Focus on building balanced habits around nutrition, sleep, and regular exercise.

30s: Balancing Responsibilities

- Work, family, and social obligations can make consistent exercise and meal planning challenging.
- Metabolism may start to slow slightly, and hormonal fluctuations can affect weight distribution.
- Prioritize time-efficient workouts, stress management, and nutrient-dense meals.

40s: Hormonal Shifts

- Perimenopause may begin, causing changes in estrogen and progesterone levels.
- Weight may accumulate around the midsection, and energy levels can fluctuate.
- Strength training, balanced nutrition, and maintaining sleep quality become crucial.

50s: Menopause and Metabolic Changes

- Post-menopause, metabolism naturally slows and muscle mass declines.
- Bone density, cardiovascular health, and joint mobility require attention.
- Focus on resistance training, calcium-rich foods, heart-healthy nutrition, and functional movement.

Beyond 60s: Maintaining Strength and Independence

Muscle loss, reduced flexibility, and chronic health conditions may affect physical activity.

Prioritize low-impact exercise, balance and mobility work, and nutrient-rich meals to support overall health and independence.

Recognizing the unique challenges of each life stage, women can adopt strategies that align with their body's changing needs, optimize weight management, and promote long-term health and vitality.

Hormones, menopause, and metabolism

Hormones play a central role in weight management, energy levels, and overall health. For women, fluctuations in hormones, particularly during perimenopause and menopause, can significantly influence metabolism, fat distribution, and appetite. Estrogen, for example, helps regulate fat storage and metabolic rate, and as levels decline during menopause, weight often accumulates around the abdomen instead of the hips and thighs. Progesterone levels also fluctuate, which can lead to bloating and temporary weight changes. Testosterone, which supports muscle mass, naturally decreases with age, slowing metabolism and reducing calorie burn. Cortisol, the stress hormone, can contribute to abdominal fat when chronically elevated due to work, family, or lifestyle stressors. At the same time, insulin sensitivity may decline over time, which can affect blood sugar control and fat storage.

To manage these hormonal shifts, it's essential to maintain lean muscle mass through regular strength training, as this supports a healthy metabolism. Focusing on a diet rich in protein and fiber can help stabilize blood sugar levels and keep you feeling full. Incorporating healthy fats, such as omega-3s from fish, flax, or walnuts, supports hormone regulation and reduces inflammation. Adequate sleep and stress management are also crucial for balancing hormones, such as cortisol. Regular cardiovascular activity helps maintain heart health and overall metabolic function. Understanding how hormones, menopause, and metabolism interact enables women to make informed lifestyle choices that maintain energy levels, support weight management, and promote long-term health as their bodies undergo changes with age.

Preventing muscle loss with age

As women age, natural changes in hormones, metabolism, and physical activity can lead to a gradual loss of muscle mass. This decline, known as sarcopenia, can affect strength, balance, and overall functional fitness, making daily activities more challenging. Preventing muscle loss is essential not only for maintaining a toned appearance but also for supporting metabolism, bone health, and long-term independence.

Incorporating regular strength training exercises is one of the most effective ways to preserve muscle. Movements that engage major muscle groups, such as squats, lunges, push-ups, and resistance work, help maintain and even build lean muscle. Adequate protein intake throughout the day further supports muscle repair and growth, while staying active through cardiovascular exercise helps maintain energy levels and overall metabolic health. Flexibility and balance work, including stretching and functional movements, complement strength training by reducing the risk of injury and improving mobility.

Prioritizing strength-building activities, balanced nutrition, and consistent physical activity, women can slow or prevent muscle loss, maintain functional independence, and continue to feel strong, capable, and confident at every stage of life.

Safe weight loss after pregnancy

Recovering and losing weight after pregnancy is a gradual process that requires patience, care, and attention to your body's changing needs. Postpartum weight loss should focus on restoring energy, supporting healing, and nurturing both mother and baby rather than quick fixes or extreme dieting. Every woman's journey is unique, and the pace of weight loss can vary depending on factors such as metabolism, activity level, breastfeeding, and overall health.

A balanced approach combines gentle physical activity with nutrient-dense meals. Strengthening exercises that target the core, back, and pelvic floor help rebuild muscle tone and support good posture, while light cardiovascular activity aids in calorie expenditure and boosts energy levels. Prioritizing protein, fiber-rich vegetables, and whole grains ensures sustained energy, supports lactation if breastfeeding, and helps manage hunger. Hydration is essential, as it supports metabolism and overall well-being.

Equally important is listening to your body and allowing ample rest. Avoid comparing your progress to others and focus on gradual, sustainable improvements. By approaching postpartum weight loss with mindfulness, consistency, and self-compassion, women can regain strength, energy, and confidence while promoting long-term health for themselves and their families.

Self-care routines for lifelong wellness

Self-care is a crucial component of maintaining health, achieving weight management, and promoting overall well-being throughout life. It extends beyond exercise and nutrition, encompassing mental, emotional, and physical practices that support long-term well-being and vitality. Prioritizing self-care helps reduce stress, improve sleep, balance hormones, and maintain energy, key factors for sustainable weight loss and overall healthy living.

Daily routines can include simple practices such as dedicating time for mindful movement, stretching, or light exercise that engages both the body and mind. Nutrition-focused self-care involves preparing balanced meals, staying hydrated, and honoring your body's hunger and fullness cues. Mental and emotional self-care can include activities such as journaling, meditation, deep breathing, or setting aside quiet moments to reflect and recharge. Social self-care, like nurturing supportive relationships, also contributes to emotional resilience and motivation.

Consistency is more important than intensity. Small, intentional daily actions compound over time, creating habits that support long-term wellness. By integrating self-care routines into your life, you cultivate a sustainable approach to health that nurtures both body and mind, empowering you to feel strong, balanced, and resilient at every stage of life.

When to consult your doctor

Knowing when to seek professional guidance is an integral part of any weight loss or wellness journey. While many lifestyle changes can be implemented safely on your own, certain situations require the expertise of a healthcare provider to ensure your approach is effective and safe.

It's wise to consult your doctor before starting a new exercise routine if you have a history of heart disease, joint issues, high blood pressure, diabetes, or any other chronic condition. Postpartum women or those recovering from surgery should also seek guidance to ensure exercises are appropriate for healing and core stability. Additionally, if you notice unexplained weight changes, persistent fatigue, or other unusual symptoms, a medical evaluation can help identify underlying causes.

Your doctor can provide personalized recommendations, monitor your progress, and help you modify nutrition or exercise plans to suit your individual health needs. Consulting a professional adds a layer of safety, confidence, and support, helping you achieve your weight loss goals while protecting your long-term health.

Staying motivated as you age

Maintaining motivation for weight loss and overall wellness can change as you move through different stages of life. Energy levels, responsibilities, and physical changes can all influence how consistently you pursue your goals. Understanding these shifts and adopting strategies to stay inspired is key to long-term success.

One of the most effective ways to stay motivated is to set realistic, meaningful goals that align with your lifestyle and personal values. Focus on improvements in strength, energy, mobility, and overall well-being rather than just the number on the scale. Celebrating small wins, tracking progress, and acknowledging your efforts can help reinforce positive habits.

Another critical factor is finding enjoyment in movement and healthy eating. Choose exercises that feel fun, social, or empowering, and create meals that nourish both body and mind. Surround yourself with supportive people, friends, family, or a community with shared goals who encourage consistency without judgment.

Be patient and compassionate with yourself. Aging is a natural process, and your body's needs evolve. Staying motivated means embracing flexibility, focusing on sustainable habits, and celebrating progress at every stage. With consistency, self-compassion, and purposeful action, you can maintain health, vitality, and confidence as you age.

CHAPTER 17

Digital Tools & Resources for Modern Weight Loss

— ∞ —

Technology has transformed the way we approach health and fitness, making it easier than ever to track progress, stay accountable, and access reliable information. This chapter examines various digital tools and resources designed to support weight loss, ranging from apps that track nutrition and exercise to wearable devices that monitor activity and sleep. By leveraging these tools, you can gain insight into your habits, set realistic goals, and receive guidance tailored to your unique needs. Understanding how to use digital resources effectively allows you to make informed decisions, stay motivated, and maintain consistent progress in your weight loss journey.

Best apps for tracking progress

Tracking your progress is a crucial part of any successful weight loss journey, and digital tools make it easier to monitor nutrition, exercise, and overall wellness. Apps can provide real-time feedback, help you set achievable goals, and keep you accountable, all from the convenience of your smartphone or tablet.

Some of the most effective apps focus on tracking food intake, calories, and macronutrients, allowing you to see patterns and make informed adjustments. Others monitor physical activity, steps, heart rate, and workout sessions to ensure you're staying active and challenging your body appropriately. Many apps also include features for tracking water intake, sleep, and mood, which can impact weight management and overall health.

By using these tools consistently, you can gain insight into your habits, celebrate small milestones, and identify areas for improvement. Choosing an app that suits your lifestyle and personal preferences can enhance motivation. It makes tracking progress simple, organized, and effective, providing you with the data you need to stay on course and achieve your weight loss goals.

Using wearables and smart devices

Wearable technology and smart devices have become powerful allies for those seeking to manage their weight and enhance overall health. Devices like fitness trackers, smartwatches, and heart rate monitors provide real-time data on steps, calories burned, sleep quality, and even stress levels, helping you make informed choices throughout the day.

By wearing a device consistently, you gain insight into your daily activity patterns, enabling you to adjust workouts, track progress, and stay accountable. Many wearables also sync with mobile apps, offering visual charts and trends that make it easier to monitor long-term progress. Beyond activity tracking, smart devices can set reminders to move, hydrate, or practice mindfulness, supporting healthy habits in small but meaningful ways.

Used thoughtfully, wearables and smart devices not only provide motivation but also help you understand your body's responses, identify patterns, and make adjustments that support sustainable weight loss. They transform abstract goals into measurable, actionable steps, keeping you engaged and empowered on your wellness journey.

Online support groups and forums

Connecting with others who share your goals can provide motivation, accountability, and practical advice throughout your weight loss journey. Online support groups and forums create a virtual community where you can share experiences, ask questions, and celebrate milestones with like-minded individuals.

These platforms offer opportunities to learn from others' successes and challenges, discover new recipes, explore effective workouts, and gain tips for overcoming obstacles. Health professionals or experienced members moderate many communities, ensuring discussions remain positive, safe, and informative. Participating in online groups can also reduce feelings of isolation, especially for those balancing busy schedules or limited access to local support networks.

Engaging with online communities allows you to receive encouragement when progress feels slow, exchange ideas for practical solutions, and build lasting connections that support your commitment to healthy habits. These virtual networks complement personal efforts, making your weight loss journey more interactive, sustainable, and rewarding.

Building your digital toolkit

Creating a personalized digital toolkit can make your weight loss journey more organized, efficient, and motivating. A digital toolkit combines apps, wearable devices, online communities, and other technology resources to track progress, monitor habits, and provide guidance tailored to your lifestyle.

Start by selecting tools that align with your specific goals and preferences. Nutrition and meal-tracking apps can help you log food, monitor macronutrients, and plan balanced meals, while wearable devices provide real-time feedback on physical activity, heart rate, and sleep. Integrating online support groups or forums adds encouragement and accountability, connecting you with a community of like-minded individuals.

The key is to choose tools that simplify your routine rather than overwhelm you. By combining these resources thoughtfully, you create a comprehensive system that supports goal setting, habit formation, and ongoing motivation. A well-structured digital toolkit empowers you to make informed choices, consistently monitor your progress, and stay engaged in your weight loss journey.

Balancing screen time with healthy habits

In today's digital world, screens are a part of almost every aspect of life, from work and social media to fitness apps and virtual support groups. While technology can support your weight loss journey, excessive screen time can contribute to sedentary behavior, disrupted sleep, and mindless snacking. Finding balance is crucial for maximizing the benefits of digital tools while maintaining overall well-being.

Start by setting boundaries for recreational screen use, and schedule dedicated time for movement, meals, and sleep without distractions. Use technology intentionally; apps, wearable's, and online communities should enhance your habits rather than replace them. For example, track workouts or meals in short, focused sessions instead of constantly scrolling, and prioritize real-world movement, such as walks, stretching, or strength exercises.

Establish screen-free routines during meals and before bedtime to support mindful eating and improve sleep quality. By balancing digital engagement with healthy, active habits, you can effectively leverage technology to support your goals without compromising your overall well-being. This thoughtful approach ensures your devices work for you, not against you, creating a sustainable environment for lifelong wellness.

Staying safe and competent online

As you leverage digital tools, apps, and online communities to support your weight loss journey, it's essential to maintain safety and privacy. Not all online information is reliable, and personal data can be vulnerable if not protected. Being cautious ensures that your experience is both productive and secure.

Begin by selecting reputable apps and platforms that have received positive reviews and clearly outlined privacy policies. Avoid sharing sensitive personal information, such as your home address or financial details, in forums or public groups. When engaging in online discussions, prioritize evidence-based advice and consult professionals before making significant changes to your nutrition, exercise, or health routines.

Be mindful of how much time you spend online. Digital tools are designed to enhance your wellness journey, not replace real-world activities or social interactions. By staying informed, verifying sources, and protecting your privacy, you can enjoy the benefits of technology while minimizing risks, creating a safe and innovative online environment that supports your long-term health goals.

CHAPTER 18

Mindset Mastery for Lasting Results

—————— ⋈ ——————

Achieving lasting weight loss and wellness is about more than just diet and exercise; it starts with the mind. Your beliefs, attitudes, and mental habits shape the choices you make daily, influencing consistency, motivation, and resilience. This chapter explores strategies to cultivate a strong, positive mindset that supports sustainable habits, helps you overcome obstacles, and empowers you to maintain results over the long term. By mastering your mindset, you can establish a solid foundation for lifelong health, confidence, and overall well-being.

Building unshakeable motivation

Motivation is the fuel that drives consistency, effort, and progress in your weight loss journey. While it naturally fluctuates, learning to cultivate and maintain unshakeable motivation can help you stay on track even during challenging times. True motivation comes from understanding your "why" and connecting it to meaningful goals that inspire you beyond the number on the scale.

To strengthen motivation, focus on small, achievable milestones that provide regular feedback and a sense of accomplishment. Celebrate these victories, whether it's completing a week of workouts, mastering a new healthy recipe, or noticing improvements in energy and strength. Surrounding yourself with supportive people, whether in person or virtually, also reinforces commitment and accountability.

It's equally important to develop strategies for when motivation dips. Techniques such as visualizing your goals, establishing daily routines, and recalling past successes can help reignite your drive and focus. By consistently reinforcing your purpose and building habits that align with your values, you create a self-sustaining system that keeps you motivated, engaged, and empowered to achieve lasting results.

Visualization and daily affirmations

Harnessing the power of your mind can significantly impact your weight loss journey. Visualization and daily affirmations are practical tools that help reinforce positive behaviors, build confidence, and maintain focus on your goals. By imagining yourself achieving milestones, such as completing a workout, preparing healthy meals, or reaching a target weight, you create a mental blueprint that encourages consistency and determination.

Daily affirmations are simple, positive statements that remind you of your strengths and reinforce healthy choices. Repeating phrases like "I am capable of achieving my goals," or "Every day I make choices that support my health" can shift your mindset from doubt to empowerment. Integrating these practices into your morning routine or before workouts strengthens mental resilience and cultivates a supportive internal dialogue.

Together, visualization and affirmations help bridge the gap between intention and action, keeping you motivated, focused, and confident in your ability to achieve lasting results. Over time, these mental practices become a natural part of your daily routine, reinforcing the habits and choices that support lifelong wellness.

Overcoming setbacks with resilience

Setbacks are a natural part of any weight loss or wellness journey. Whether it's missing a workout, indulging at a social event, or experiencing slower-than-expected results, these moments don't define your progress—they offer opportunities to learn and grow. Developing resilience helps you navigate obstacles without losing motivation or confidence.

Resilient individuals approach challenges with a solution-focused mindset. Instead of dwelling on mistakes, they analyze what led to the setback, adjust their strategies, and take proactive steps to get back on track. This might mean planning meals ahead of a busy week, incorporating shorter workouts when time is limited, or reframing negative self-talk into encouraging thoughts.

Building resilience also involves self-compassion. Recognize that perfection isn't required and that progress comes from consistent effort over time. By maintaining perspective, staying flexible, and using challenges as learning experiences, you strengthen both your mindset and your commitment. Overcoming setbacks with resilience ensures that temporary obstacles become stepping stones, supporting sustainable weight loss and long-term health.

Journaling for accountability

Journaling is a powerful tool to maintain accountability and clarity throughout your weight loss journey. By putting your goals, progress, and reflections on paper, you create a tangible record of your efforts and achievements. This practice helps you track patterns in eating, exercise, sleep, and mood, providing insight into what works best for your body and lifestyle.

Daily or weekly journaling can include recording workouts, meals, water intake, energy levels, and emotions tied to food or activity. Reflecting on successes and challenges allows you to celebrate progress and identify areas for improvement without judgment. Writing also encourages mindfulness, making you more aware of decisions and helping you stay focused on long-term goals.

Journaling serves as a motivational tool. Reviewing past entries can remind you of your resilience during difficult periods and reinforce your commitment to healthy habits. Over time, this practice enhances self-awareness, cultivates discipline, and fosters a sense of accountability that supports sustainable weight loss and promotes lifelong wellness.

Stress relief for consistency

Stress can be one of the most significant barriers to maintaining healthy habits and consistent progress in a weight loss journey. Elevated stress levels often lead to emotional eating, disrupted sleep patterns, and a decrease in motivation to exercise. Learning to manage stress effectively is crucial for achieving long-term success and promoting overall well-being.

Incorporating stress-relief practices into your daily routine can help you stay consistent with your goals. Techniques such as deep breathing, meditation, or yoga calm the nervous system, reduce tension, and enhance focus. Regular physical activity, even in short sessions, not only supports fitness but also acts as a natural stress reliever by releasing endorphins. Engaging in hobbies, spending time in nature, or connecting with supportive friends and family also contributes to emotional balance.

By managing stress proactively, you create an environment that fosters healthy habits. Consistency becomes easier when your mind and body are calm, focused, and energized, allowing you to navigate life's challenges without compromising your weight loss or wellness objectives.

Future-proofing your success

Sustainable weight loss and wellness are not just about achieving short-term goals; they are about establishing habits and routines that last a lifetime. Future-proofing your success means developing strategies, mindsets, and behaviors that enable you to maintain progress, adapt to changes, and continue thriving despite life's challenges.

This involves cultivating a strong foundation of healthy eating, consistent physical activity, and mindful self-care, while also remaining flexible when circumstances shift. Tracking progress, reflecting on successes and setbacks, and adjusting routines as needed ensures that your approach evolves with your body and lifestyle. Maintaining motivation through visualization, goal setting, and support systems further reinforces long-term commitment.

Thinking beyond immediate results and prioritizing habits that can be sustained for years, you equip yourself with the tools, knowledge, and mindset to maintain a healthy weight, preserve strength and energy, and enjoy a balanced, vibrant life well into the future. This forward-looking approach turns your current achievements into lasting wellness.

Conclusion

Achieving lasting weight loss and wellness is a journey that goes far beyond the numbers on a scale. It encompasses a holistic approach that combines balanced nutrition, consistent movement, mindful habits, and a resilient mindset. Throughout this book, you've explored strategies for understanding your unique physiology, managing emotional and social challenges, creating sustainable routines, and leveraging tools and resources to support your goals.

The key to long-term success is consistency, patience, and self-compassion. There will be challenges, setbacks, and busy periods, but every small step you take contributes to your overall progress. By focusing on building healthy habits, listening to your body, and nurturing both physical and mental well-being, you create a foundation that supports weight management and vitality for life.

This journey is uniquely yours. Celebrate your achievements, learn from obstacles, and continue to adapt your approach as your needs and life circumstances change. With knowledge, dedication, and the mindset tools you've gained, you are equipped to maintain your results, embrace a healthier lifestyle, and enjoy the confidence, energy, and strength that come with lifelong wellness.

www.ingramcontent.com/pod-product-compliance
Lightning Source LLC
Chambersburg PA
CBHW062052270326
41931CB00013B/3045